Athletic Fuel

Nutrition Science Explained for Athletes

Written by Jon Ramsey

Published by Cornell-David Publishing House

Index

1. Fuelling Athletic Performance

1.1 Understanding the Importance of Nutrition in Athletic Performance

A well-designed training program is essential for athletes to reach the pinnacle of their sport, but what sets one athlete apart from another is often their attention to nutrition. Sports nutrition plays a vital role in optimizing every aspect of athletic performance – it affects an athlete's energy levels, body composition, strength, recovery, and overall health. In this section, we will explain the fundamentals of sports nutrition, why it is important and provide evidence-based guidance on how to fuel athletic performance before, during, and after physical activity.

1.1.1 Macronutrients: The Building Blocks of Athletic Fuel

The three primary macronutrients that act as sources of energy for the body are carbohydrates, fats, and proteins. Here is a brief overview of their importance to an athlete's performance:

- **Carbohydrates:** The primary and preferred energy source of the body, especially during high-intensity activities. They provide glucose, which can be stored as glycogen in the muscles and liver for later use. Athletes with adequate glycogen stores will perform better in their training and competitions, experience reduced fatigue, and recover more rapidly between training sessions.

- **Fats:** The most concentrated source of energy and a key component of long-duration training or endurance sports, where the body is required to use fat for fuel when glycogen stores are low. In addition to energy provision, fats also play a vital role in hormone production, vitamin absorption, cell membrane health, and inflammation regulation.
- **Proteins:** Although not a primary source of energy, proteins are crucial for muscle growth, maintenance, and repair. They also support immune function, hormone production, and other physiological mechanisms essential to an athlete's health and performance. Consuming optimal amounts and types of protein can help athletes adapt better to training stimuli, recover faster, and reduce the risk of injuries.

1.1.2 Micronutrients: Supporting Energy Production and Overall Health

Vitamins and minerals, collectively referred to as micronutrients, may not provide energy like macronutrients, but they play a crucial role in various physiological processes essential to an athlete's health and performance. Maintaining the right balance of micronutrients is vital to support energy production, oxygen transport, bone health, immune function, and metabolism.

Some key micronutrients of importance for athletes include:

- **Iron:** A key mineral involved in oxygen transportation, playing a critical role in endurance events. Low iron levels can lead to anemia, which compromises oxygen transportation and results in decreased athletic performance.
- **Calcium and Vitamin D:** Crucial nutrients for maintaining bone density and reducing the risk of

stress fractures, which can sideline athletes for months. Vitamin D also plays a role in immune health and muscle function.

- **Magnesium:** Involved in energy production, muscle contraction, and bone health, magnesium is crucial for athletes. Insufficient magnesium intake may cause muscle cramps, weakness, and fatigue.
- **B-vitamins:** Their importance is paramount, especially for athletes, as they are involved in energy production and metabolism, breaking down carbohydrates and fats into usable energy.

1.1.3 Hydration: The Key to Peak Performance

Staying adequately hydrated is essential for overall health and athletic performance, as even mild dehydration can adversely affect an athlete's performance. Water is involved in many physiological processes, from delivering nutrients to cells and regulating body temperature to lubricating joints and dissolving minerals and vitamins necessary for optimal body function.

Athletes should monitor their fluid intake and adjust their hydration strategies based on factors such as body size, climate, training intensity, and sweat rate. Dehydration not only reduces performance by affecting factors such as muscle strength, reaction time, and decision-making but- if left unchecked- can also lead to heat-related illnesses, which can be life-threatening.

1.1.4 Strategies for Nutrient Timing and Personalization

An athlete's optimal nutrition plan is not a one-size-fits-all approach; it requires customization based on factors such as age, gender, body composition, sport-specific demands, training goals, and individual preferences. Proper nutrient timing, especially around training or competition sessions, can optimize energy availability, recovery, and adaptation.

Key factors to consider in nutrient timing strategies include:

- **Pre-exercise:** Consuming a meal or snack rich in carbohydrates, moderate in protein, and low in fat can help fuel subsequent athletic performance and prevent excessive hunger during activity.
- **During exercise:** Staying hydrated and consuming carbohydrates during prolonged activities can help maintain performance by providing a steady supply of glucose, preserving glycogen stores, and delaying the onset of fatigue.
- **Post-exercise:** Consuming a combination of carbohydrates and proteins in a specific ratio (3:1) within a crucial window of time post-exercise (~30 minutes) can jump-start the recovery process, replenish glycogen stores, and repair muscle tissue, preparing the athlete for the next bout of training or competition.

In the coming chapters, we will expand on these principles and delve deeper into crafting nutrition plans tailored to individual needs and athletic goals. Armed with this knowledge, athletes can optimize their fueling strategies, enhance their performance, and gain a competitive edge.

1.1 Understanding the Role of Nutrition in Athletic Performance

In the realm of athletics, nutrition plays an essential role in optimizing performance, promoting recovery, and supporting long-term health. As part of a comprehensive training plan, a well-balanced diet provides a strong foundation for athletes seeking to push their physical limits and achieve their specific performance goals. In this section, we will explore the science behind sports nutrition and its influence on athletic performance.

1.1.1 Macronutrients: The Building Blocks of Athletic Performance

To gain an understanding of sports nutrition, it is vital to first comprehend the role of macronutrients - the primary components of our diet responsible for providing the energy required for various bodily functions, including athletic performance. There are three primary macronutrients: carbohydrates, fats, and proteins, each with its unique properties and roles in the body.

Carbohydrates: Often the primary fuel source for athletes, carbohydrates (carbs) are broken down into glucose molecules, which are then utilized for energy or stored in the form of glycogen in muscles and the liver. During exercise, particularly high-intensity or endurance training, muscle glycogen stores are rapidly depleted. Consuming an adequate amount of carbohydrates before and after exercise can help replenish these stores, thus optimizing performance and recovery.

Fats: While carbohydrates are the body's preferred energy source, fats also play a crucial role in fueling endurance and lower-intensity activities. Fats are broken down into fatty acids, which can then be used to produce energy when carbohydrate availability is limited, particularly during prolonged exercise. In addition, fats are essential for hormonal regulation, cellular function, and nutrient absorption.

Proteins: Proteins are the building blocks of all tissues in the body, including muscles. They are made up of amino acids, which are critically involved in processes such as muscle synthesis, recovery, and repair. For athletes, consuming an adequate amount of protein throughout the day is essential for maintaining, repairing, and building lean muscle mass, ultimately supporting athletic performance.

1.1.2 Micronutrients and Fluids: Supporting Optimal Function

In addition to macronutrients, micronutrients (vitamins and minerals) and fluids also contribute to optimal athletic performance by supporting various physiological processes and maintaining overall health.

Vitamins: Vitamins are essential organic compounds required in small quantities for optimal bodily function. They play crucial roles in various physiological processes necessary for athletic performance, such as energy production, bone health, immune function, and antioxidant protection.

Minerals: Minerals are inorganic compounds needed for various bodily functions, such as electrolyte regulation, muscle function, bone maintenance, and immune support. Athletes may require greater amounts of certain minerals due to increased demands, losses through sweat, or other sports-related factors.

Fluids: Proper hydration is a critical component of athletic performance, as fluids are necessary for maintaining blood volume, temperature regulation, and cellular function. Dehydration can negatively affect strength, endurance, power, and cognitive function, ultimately stifering athletic potential.

1.1.3 Individualized Nutrition Strategies: Catering to the Unique Needs of Athletes

It is important to acknowledge that individual athletes possess differing nutritional requirements based on factors such as sport type, training volume and intensity, body composition, and personal preferences. As a result, sports nutrition strategies should be tailored to the individual in order to optimize performance, recovery, and overall health.

Sport Type: The nutritional needs of an athlete will vary depending on the specific sport and its corresponding energy requirements. For example, endurance sports such as marathon running typically demand greater carbohydrate intake to fuel prolonged bouts of exercise, whereas strength and power sports, such as weightlifting, may necessitate greater protein consumption to support muscle repair and growth.

Training Volume and Intensity: The amount and intensity of training an athlete participates in will influence their nutritional needs. An athlete engaged in high-volume or intense training sessions will require increased amounts of macronutrients, micronutrients, and fluids to support energy replenishment, recovery, and health.

Body Composition Goals: An athlete's body composition goals may also influence their nutrition strategies. For example, an individual seeking to reduce body fat may adjust their macronutrient ratios and caloric intake according to their unique weight loss targets.

Personal Preferences: Lastly, personal preferences, dietary restrictions, and cultural or religious practices should be considered when creating tailored nutrition plans for athletes in order to promote adherence and long-term success.

In conclusion, a thorough understanding of the science behind sports nutrition is fundamental for athletes striving for optimal performance, recovery, and health. By cultivating awareness of the primary components of diet, acknowledging individual nutrition needs, and implementing tailored strategies, athletes can effectively fuel their bodies to propel them towards greater success in their chosen sport.

1.1 Fuelling Athletic Performance: The Importance of Sports Nutrition

Athletes, whether professional or amateur, often overlook a crucial aspect of their overall performance and well-being: **sports nutrition**. While many people might be aware of the importance of proper nutrition, they often don't understand how it directly impacts athletic performance. The old saying, *you are what you eat*, holds especially true for athletes, as the nutrients they consume serve as the fuel for their activity. In this chapter, we will discuss the key principles of sports nutrition and explore how to optimize an athlete's diet for better performance, recovery, and overall health.

1.1.1 Macronutrients: The Building Blocks of Athletic Performance

Macronutrients are the nutrients required by the body in large quantities to produce energy and maintain essential physiological functions. There are three main macronutrients: **carbohydrates**, **protein** and **fats**.

Carbohydrates

Carbohydrates are the primary fuel source for an athlete's body. They are broken down into glucose, which is then stored in the liver and muscles as glycogen. The body relies on this glycogen during both aerobic and anaerobic activities to produce the energy needed for muscles to contract, making carbohydrate consumption essential for peak performance.

There are two main types of carbohydrates: complex and simple. Complex carbohydrates (such as whole grains, starchy vegetables, and legumes) are ideal for sustained energy release, while simple carbohydrates (like fruit and sports gels) provide a quick energy boost. Athletes should consume a mix of complex and simple carbohydrates according to the specific needs of their sport.

Protein

While carbohydrates are essential for providing immediate energy during physical activity, protein's primary role is to repair and build muscle tissue damaged during exercise. Consuming adequate protein is essential for athletes, as it helps to maintain and increase muscle mass, which can directly impact performance.

Moreover, protein plays a crucial role in numerous other physiological processes, such as immune function, hormone production, and fluid balance. Athletes should consume a variety of high-quality protein sources like lean meats, fish, poultry, dairy products, legumes, and certain plant-based proteins.

Fats

Fats are the most energy-dense macronutrient, supplying 9 calories per gram compared to 4 calories per gram for carbohydrates and protein. They serve as an important source of stored energy for exercise, especially during low-intensity and prolonged activity. Additionally, fats are vital for proper hormone production, brain function, and nutrient absorption.

Fats can be divided into two primary categories: saturated and unsaturated fats. Unsaturated fats, including monounsaturated and polyunsaturated fats (e.g., omega-3 and omega-6 fatty acids), are considered healthier options and should make up the majority of an athlete's fat intake. These can be found in foods such as avocados, nuts, seeds, fish, and plant-based oils.

1.1.2 Micronutrients: Supporting Performance and Health

While macronutrients provide the body with energy and building blocks for tissue repair, micronutrients play a critical role in various physiological processes that support athletic performance, recovery, and overall health. Micronutrients include vitamins and minerals, which help the body to function optimally during training and competition.

Key micronutrients for athletes include:

- **Iron**: vital for oxygen transport and energy production
- **Calcium**: essential for bone health and muscle contraction
- **Magnesium**: crucial for muscle function, energy metabolism, and nerve function
- **Vitamin D**: supports bone health and immune function
- **B Vitamins**: involved in energy production and the formation of red blood cells

- **Antioxidants**: (e.g., Vitamin C, Vitamin E, and selenium) protect cells from damage and support immune function

Athletes should consume a well-balanced diet rich in fruits, vegetables, whole grains, lean proteins, and healthy fats to ensure they receive adequate amounts of these essential micronutrients.

1.1.3 Hydration: Fluid Balance for Optimal Performance

Proper hydration is crucial for athletic performance. An athlete's body can lose significant amounts of fluid through sweat, urine, and respiration, leading to dehydration. Dehydration can impair both physical and mental performance, increasing the risk of injury and heat-related illnesses like heat stroke.

To maintain optimal hydration, athletes should consume fluids before, during, and after exercise. The American College of Sports Medicine (ACSM) recommends that athletes consume 16-20 ounces of fluid (typically water or sports drinks with electrolytes) 2-3 hours prior to exercise, 7-10 ounces every 10-20 minutes during exercise, and approximately 20-24 ounces of fluid for every one pound of body weight lost during exercise.

In addition to water, sports drinks containing electrolytes such as sodium, potassium, and magnesium can help to offset losses incurred during intense or prolonged activity. These electrolytes play a critical role in maintaining fluid balance and preventing muscle cramps.

1.1.4 Individualization and Periodization: Tailoring Nutrition to Your Needs

While the principles of sports nutrition remain constant, each athlete's specific nutritional needs may vary based on factors such as body composition, fitness level, training load, and personal goals. It is essential for athletes to individualize their nutrition plans according to their unique circumstances and track their progress over time.

Moreover, an athlete's nutritional needs may change throughout different phases of the training cycle, known as periodization. As training load and intensity fluctuate, so should the macronutrient distribution to ensure proper fueling and recovery.

In conclusion, a solid foundation in sports nutrition is essential for maximizing athletic performance, optimizing recovery, and promoting overall health. By understanding the fundamental principles of macronutrients, micronutrients, hydration, and individualization, athletes can create a nutrition plan that fuels their performance and supports their long-term athletic goals.

1.1 The Importance of Nutrition for Athletic Performance

In the world of sports and athletic activities, the role of nutrition cannot be overstated. Nutrition essentially functions as the foundation upon which an athlete's performance and overall well-being is built. In order for athletes to achieve optimal performance levels, their bodies need the correct balance of nutrients, including carbohydrates, proteins, fats, vitamins, minerals, and water. Without proper nutrition, an athlete's health, strength, and overall athletic abilities may be compromised. Consequently, understanding the science of sports nutrition and its application to individualized training programs is crucial for athletes to enhance performance, prevent injuries, and ensure a long, vital athletic career.

1.1.1 The Three Macronutrients: Carbohydrates, Proteins, and Fats

The primary components of nutrition that greatly influence athletic performance are the three macronutrients: carbohydrates, proteins, and fats.

- **Carbohydrates**: As the main source of energy for most athletic activities, carbohydrates play an indispensable role in fueling athletic performance. Carbs are broken down into glucose, which is then stored in the muscles and liver as glycogen. During physical activities, the body converts glycogen back into glucose to provide the energy needed for muscle contractions. Depending on an athlete's specific energy requirements, carbohydrate intake should be individualized and appropriately timed.
- **Proteins**: Proteins are essential building blocks for the growth, repair, and maintenance of muscle tissues. They comprise amino acids, the basic units that form various body structures such as muscles, bones, tendons, and ligaments. An adequate protein intake is crucial for athletes, as it supports muscle recovery, reduces muscle breakdown, and assists in muscle growth. The amount of protein an athlete needs depends on factors such as sport type, training volume, and individual requirements.

- **Fats**: Fats serve as a vital energy source, particularly for endurance athletes who engage in longer and less intense physical activities. In addition to providing energy, fats play essential roles in the body, including cellular function, insulation, hormone regulation, and nutrient absorption. While fat is essential for health and performance, it is important for athletes to focus on consuming healthy fats, such as monounsaturated and polyunsaturated fats, while minimizing the consumption of unhealthy trans fats and limiting saturated fats.

1.1.2 Micronutrients: Vitamins and Minerals

In addition to macronutrients, micronutrients, or vitamins and minerals, are necessary for optimal athletic performance. Although required in smaller amounts compared to macronutrients, micronutrients are essential for various physiological functions, such as energy production, muscle function, and immune system support.

Some key micronutrients that play a significant role in athletic performance include:

- **Vitamin D**: This fat-soluble vitamin is important for calcium absorption, which in turn plays a crucial role in bone health and muscle function. It has been suggested that vitamin D may also contribute to improving muscle strength and reducing inflammation.
- **Iron**: Iron is essential for oxygen transport within the body, as it is a key component of hemoglobin, the molecule responsible for binding oxygen to red blood cells. Athletes, particularly endurance athletes, face a

higher risk for iron deficiency due to the increased demand for oxygen delivery to working muscles.

- **Calcium**: This mineral is well-known for its importance in bone health, but it also plays a crucial role in muscle function and normal nerve conduction. Athletes with inadequate calcium intake may face a higher risk for stress fractures and disturbances in muscle function.
- **Magnesium**: Magnesium is involved in multiple physiological processes, including energy production, protein synthesis, and nerve and muscle function. Some research has indicated that higher magnesium intake may be associated with improved athletic performance.

1.1.3 Hydration

Water is an essential element that holds various functions in the body, including nutrient transport, waste removal, body temperature regulation, and joint lubrication. Maintaining proper hydration levels is critical for athletes, as even mild dehydration can lead to decreased performance, increased fatigue, and a higher risk of injuries. Athletes should develop individualized hydration strategies based on factors such as body size, sweat rates, environmental conditions, and exercise duration and intensity.

1.1.4 Nutrient Timing

While ensuring an adequate intake of carbohydrates, proteins, fats, and micronutrients is essential for athletes, paying attention to nutrient timing and the specific demands of their training regimen can further help maximize athletic performance.

- **Pre-Exercise Nutrition**: Providing the body with fuel before exercise can help optimize energy levels, reduce muscle protein breakdown, and enhance physical and mental performance. Athletes should aim at consuming a meal rich in carbohydrates, moderate in protein, and low in fat and fiber approximately 2-4 hours before exercising to avoid gastrointestinal discomfort.
- **During-Exercise Nutrition**: Proper nutrition during exercise can help maintain energy levels, reduce fatigue, and support an athlete in sustaining their effort. Depending on the duration and intensity of the activity, athletes may need to consume fluids, electrolytes, and carbohydrates (in the form of easily digestible sports drinks or gels) to support their performance.
- **Post-Exercise Nutrition**: The period after exercise is critical for athletes, as it is their opportunity to refuel their bodies and support muscle recovery and adaptation. A well-rounded post-exercise meal or snack should include carbohydrates to replenish glycogen stores, proteins to promote muscle repair and growth, and fluids and electrolytes to replace the water and minerals lost through sweat.

Understanding the science of sports nutrition and how it influences athletic performance allows athletes to optimize their diet and make informed choices about the foods they consume before, during, and after their training sessions. By focusing on the quality and timing of their meals, athletes will better prepare their bodies for the demands of exercise, ultimately enhancing their performance and long-term success in their chosen sport.

1.1 Fuelling Athletic Performance: The Role of Nutrition in Sport

Athletic performance undeniably relies on a combination of skill, dedication, and discipline. Behind the scenes, however, it is essential to consider the foundational role that nutrition plays in fuelling this performance. While it may often be overlooked compared to training, recovery, and mental preparation, sports nutrition is vital in supporting an athlete's growth, health, and ability to recover from injury or intense workouts. With a myriad of information on this topic, it can be challenging to navigate the waters and understand what truly benefits athletic bodies. This section aims to break down the science behind sports nutrition and how it can be applied to enhance your training and optimize your athletic potential.

1.1.1 Macronutrients: The Building Blocks of Optimal Performance

Macronutrients, comprising carbohydrates, proteins, and fats, are the primary nutrients responsible for providing energy and fuel to perform daily tasks and engage in athletic activities. Here is a brief overview of each macronutrient's role in sports nutrition:

- **Carbohydrates:** Often touted as the body's primary energy source, carbohydrates fuel high-intensity activities via glycogen stores in the muscles and liver. Due to the body's limited storage capacity for glycogen, it is essential for athletes to consume adequate carbohydrates to replenish these stores and prevent fatigue during training or competition. Complex carbs such as whole grains, fruits, and vegetables are ideal sources due to their steady release of energy.

- **Proteins:** Integral for building and repairing muscle tissue, proteins are composed of amino acids, the building blocks for many essential functions within the body. Adequate protein intake is crucial for athletes as it supports lean muscle mass, immune function, and injury recovery. Options such as lean meats, fish, dairy, legumes, and plant-based proteins are excellent choices for athletes to incorporate into their diet.
- **Fats:** Fats play an essential role in energy production, vitamin absorption, and the maintenance of cell membranes. Because fats are more energy-dense than carbohydrates, they are the primary source of fuel for lower intensity activities. Including a balance of unsaturated, saturated, and polyunsaturated fat sources such as avocados, nuts, seeds, and omega-rich fish can support overall health and athletic performance.

1.1.2 Micronutrients: The Tiny Helpers in Athletic Success

While macronutrients are the central components of any diet, micronutrients (vitamins and minerals) play a pivotal role in optimizing athletic performance as they support many essential processes within the body. Deficiency in micronutrients can lead to sluggishness, impaired recovery, and other unwanted side effects that impede performance. Some of the most critical micronutrients for athletes include:

- **Vitamins:** B-group vitamins for energy metabolism, vitamin C for its role in collagen synthesis and

antioxidant properties, and vitamin D for muscle and bone health.
- **Minerals:** Iron for oxygen transport, calcium and magnesium for healthy bone and muscle function, and zinc for immune support and protein synthesis.

1.1.3 Hydration: The Unsung Hero in Sport Performance

The importance of proper hydration extends far beyond quenching thirst. It is the essence of many bodily processes, making it crucial for overall wellbeing and athletic performance. Poor hydration can lead to a drop in blood volume, resulting in reduced oxygen and nutrient delivery to working muscles, impaired body temperature regulation, and compromised cognitive function. Athletes should consistently monitor fluid intake, aiming to consume water and electrolytes regularly to maintain performance levels and prevent dehydration.

1.1.4 Nutrient Timing: The Secret Sauce for Performance and Recovery

The timing of nutrition intake can play an essential role in optimizing performance and recovery. Pre-workout nutrition should provide enough fuel without causing discomfort or sluggishness during the activity. Meals high in carbohydrates, moderate in protein, and low in fat are ideal to ensure readily available energy and minimal digestion time.

Post-workout nutrition is crucial for replenishing glycogen stores and facilitating muscle repair. Consuming carbohydrates and proteins immediately following a workout can enhance recovery, promote muscle growth and prepare the body for subsequent training sessions.

1.1.5 Individualized Nutrition: The Key to Unlocking Peak Performance

While the fundamental principles of sports nutrition apply to all athletes, customization based on individual needs is key. Factors like age, gender, body composition, training goals, and cultural dietary preferences must be considered when planning an athlete's diet. Consultation with a sports nutrition professional can guide athletes in tailoring their nutrition plan to align with their unique needs and goals.

In conclusion, sports nutrition plays an indispensable role in fuelling athletic performance. By understanding the science behind macronutrients, micronutrients, hydration, and nutrient timing, athletes can optimize their diet to support their training and performance goals. Ultimately, recognizing the importance of individualized nutrition will unlock the gates to peak performance, health, and wellbeing.

2. The Role of Macronutrients: Carbohydrates, Proteins, and Fats

2.1 Carbohydrates: The Athlete's Primary Fuel Source

Carbohydrates can be considered the most important macronutrient for athletes, as they serve as the primary fuel source for physical activity, especially during high-intensity exercise.

2.1.1 Types of Carbohydrates

There are three types of carbohydrates:

1. Monosaccharides - simple sugars consisting of a single molecule, such as glucose, fructose, and galactose.
2. Disaccharides - Two monosaccharides linked together. Examples include sucrose, lactose, and maltose.
3. Polysaccharides - Complex carbohydrates formed by long chains of monosaccharide units. Notable examples are starch, glycogen, and fiber.

From an athlete's perspective, our primary focus should be on glucose, as it is the main carbohydrate that provides energy for bodily functions and sport performance.

2.1.2 The Importance of Carbohydrates for Athletes

Carbohydrates are vital for athletic performance for several reasons:

1. **Energy production**: Carbohydrates are the body's primary and quickest source of energy. The body breaks down carbohydrates into glucose, which is used to fuel exercising muscles and other organs.
2. **Glycogen storage**: The body stores carbohydrates in the form of glycogen in both the liver and muscles. Liver glycogen primarily helps to maintain blood sugar levels, while muscle glycogen acts as a direct energy source for working muscles during exercise.
3. **Supports high-intensity exercise**: During high-intensity exercise, such as sprinting or powerlifting, carbohydrates are the primary fuel source. The body can produce ATP (adenosine triphosphate) from carbohydrates faster than from fats or proteins, which is crucial for maintaining the intensity of the activity.

2.1.3 Carbohydrate Intake Recommendations for Athletes

Carbohydrate intake recommendations for athletes depend on various factors, including the type, duration, and intensity of the exercise, as well as the athlete's personal goals, such as muscle building, optimal performance, or endurance.

General guidelines for carbohydrate intake are as follows:

- **Recreational athletes**: 5-7 grams of carbohydrates per kilogram of body weight per day
- **Endurance athletes**: 7-10 grams of carbohydrates per kilogram of body weight per day

- **Ultra-endurance athletes**: 10-12 grams of carbohydrates per kilogram of body weight per day

It's important to note that these recommendations may change based on the athlete's training schedule, nutritional goals, and caloric needs.

2.1.4 Timing of Carbohydrate Intake

To maximize athletic performance and recovery, athletes should consider both the timing and quantity of carbohydrate intake.

1. **Before exercise**: Consuming a carbohydrate-rich meal or snack 1-4 hours before exercise ensures that sufficient glycogen stores are available for optimal performance. This can help to prevent "hitting the wall" or "bonking", which occurs when glycogen stores are depleted, leading to a significant decline in energy levels.
2. **During exercise**: For prolonged and high-intensity training sessions or events (60-90 minutes or longer), consuming quick-release carbohydrates can help maintain blood glucose levels and boost endurance.
3. **After exercise**: Replenishing glycogen stores after exercise is crucial for proper recovery, especially if the athlete plans to train or compete again within the next 24 hours. Consuming carbohydrates within 30 minutes to 2 hours post-exercise is considered optimal for glycogen resynthesis.

2.1.5 Quality of Carbohydrates

Selecting high-quality carbohydrate sources is as important as consuming an appropriate quantity. Athletes should prioritize complex carbohydrates, like whole grains, legumes, fruits, and vegetables, while limiting simple sugars and refined carbohydrates, such as candy, pastries, and white bread. Complex carbohydrates provide a more steady and prolonged source of energy, beneficial for both performance and recovery, as well as additional nutrients, like fiber, vitamins, and minerals essential for overall health.

In summary, carbohydrates play a crucial role as the primary fuel source for athletes. Proper intake, timing, and quality of carbohydrates can significantly impact athletic performance and help athletes reach their full potential.

2.1 Carbohydrates: Energy Powerhouses for Athletes

Carbohydrates serve as the primary and most efficient source of energy for athletes during physical exertion. They are classified into two major types: simple carbohydrates (or sugars) and complex carbohydrates (or starches and fibers).

2.1.1 Simple Carbohydrates

Simple carbohydrates, also known as sugars, are quickly broken down and absorbed into the bloodstream. They provide the body with an almost instant energy boost. Common sources of simple carbohydrates include fruits, milk, honey, and table sugar. While these sugars provide a quick burst of energy, they may not last long, possibly leading to a crash, commonly known as a "sugar high" followed by a "sugar crash."

2.1.2 Complex Carbohydrates

Complex carbohydrates, as the name suggests, have a more complex structure compared to simple carbohydrates. This complexity slows down their digestion and absorption, providing a more sustained and steady release of energy.

Complex carbohydrates are found in whole grains, legumes, and vegetables. These sources also provide essential vitamins, minerals, and fibers, making them a crucial component of an athlete's diet.

For athletes, it is necessary to consume a combination of both simple and complex carbohydrates. Simple carbs provide the quick energy needed during exercise, while complex carbs offer more stable energy levels to prevent a crash or to aid in recovery after exertion.

2.1.3 Glycogen: Essential Storage Form of Carbohydrates

When carbohydrates are consumed, the body breaks them down into glucose, its primary energy source. Excess glucose gets stored in the liver and muscles in the form of glycogen. During intense physical activity, the body relies on glycogen reserves to sustain energy levels. Once glycogen stores are depleted, physical performance may suffer, causing fatigue, reduced endurance, and compromised strength. Therefore, maintaining adequate glycogen reserves is critical for athletes, especially those engaged in endurance sports like marathon running, cycling, or swimming.

To optimize glycogen stores, athletes are recommended to consume high-quality carbohydrates in sufficient quantities. A widely accepted guideline is to consume between 6 to 10 grams of carbohydrates per kilogram of body weight daily, depending on the intensity and duration of training. For example, a 70 kg endurance athlete should aim for 420 to 700 grams of carbohydrates per day.

2.1.4 Carbohydrate Timing for Optimal Performance

To maximize glycogen stores and ensure proper energy levels, carbohydrate consumption should be timed strategically. Key time periods for carbohydrate consumption include:

- **Pre-Exercise:** Consuming carbohydrates 3-4 hours before exercise can help boost energy and glycogen stores. Aim for a meal that is high in complex carbohydrates, moderate in protein, and low in fat. If necessary, a small snack containing simple carbohydrates can be consumed 30-60 minutes before exercise to provide an extra energy boost.
- **During Exercise:** For endurance events lasting longer than an hour, consuming 30-60 grams of carbohydrates per hour can significantly improve performance by maintaining blood glucose levels and delaying the depletion of glycogen stores.
- **Post-Exercise:** It is essential to replace lost glycogen stores after an intense workout. Consuming carbohydrates within the first 30 minutes to 2 hours after exercise is ideal for replenishing glycogen reserves and promoting recovery. Aim for a 31 or 41 ratio of carbohydrates-to-protein for optimal glycogen synthesis and muscle repair.

2.2 Proteins: Building Blocks for Muscle Growth and Repair

Proteins are the structural component of nearly all body tissues, including muscles, tendons, and ligaments. They consist of long chains of amino acids, which are the body's building blocks. Proper protein intake is crucial for muscle growth, repair, and maintenance.

Athletes, particularly those involved in strength and power sports, have higher protein requirements than sedentary individuals. Adequate protein intake aids in muscle hypertrophy (growth), prevents muscle breakdown during exercise, and promotes muscle recovery after physical exertion. The American College of Sports Medicine and the American Dietetic Association recommend an intake of 1.2 to 2 grams of protein per kilogram of body weight daily, depending on the intensity and type of training. For example, an 80 kg strength athlete should aim for 96 to 160 grams of protein per day.

It is critical for athletes to consume a variety of protein sources, both animal and plant-based, to obtain all of the essential amino acids required for optimal muscle function. Foods rich in high-quality proteins include lean meats, fish, poultry, dairy products, beans, lentils, and soy products. Consuming protein with carbohydrates post-exercise can further enhance muscle recovery and glycogen synthesis.

2.3 Fats: Essential for Optimal Health and Performance

Fats are an essential macronutrient, playing a critical role in an athlete's diet. Fats provide energy, assist in the absorption of essential nutrients, protect vital organs, and regulate hormones.

Fats are categorized into three main types: saturated, unsaturated, and trans fats. Athletes should prioritize consuming unsaturated fats, which are found in foods such as olive oil, avocados, nuts, and fatty fish. Unsaturated fats help reduce inflammation, which is vital for athletic recovery, and maintain healthy cholesterol levels.

While saturated fats have been negatively associated with cardiovascular health, they should not be entirely excluded from an athlete's diet. However, moderation is key when consuming saturated fats, which are typically found in animal products and full-fat dairy. Trans fats, on the other hand, should be avoided as they are associated with increased inflammation and cardiovascular risk.

Athletes should aim to consume between 20 to 35% of their total daily caloric intake from fats. However, it is important to remember that fats are more calorie-dense than carbohydrates and proteins, with 9 calories per gram, compared to 4 calories per gram for the latter two. Therefore, portion control is essential when consuming fats.

In conclusion, a well-rounded diet that includes adequate amounts of carbohydrates, proteins, and fats is crucial for athletes to optimize their performance, promote recovery, and maintain overall health. By understanding the roles of these macronutrients and tailoring their intake based on their individual needs, athletes can fuel their bodies effectively and achieve their performance goals.

2.1 Carbohydrates: The Primary Fuel for Athletes

Carbohydrates serve as the main energy source for athletes, particularly those involved in high-intensity and endurance sports. When consumed, carbohydrates are broken down into glucose, which is then transported and utilized by the body or stored as glycogen in the liver and muscles. During exercise, these glycogen stores are crucial as they are the primary fuel source for working muscles.

2.1.1 Types of Carbohydrates

Carbohydrates can be categorized into simple and complex forms based on their structure and digestion speed.

- **Simple Carbohydrates** - These are composed of one or two sugar molecules (monosaccharides and disaccharides) and are quickly absorbed and utilized by the body. Examples include fructose found in fruits and lactose in dairy products. Simple sugars can be particularly useful for athletes needing a rapid energy source during or immediately after a workout.
- **Complex Carbohydrates** - Consisting of long chains of sugar molecules (polysaccharides), complex carbohydrates take longer to digest, resulting in sustained energy release over time. Foods like whole grains, legumes, and starchy vegetables are a primary source of complex carbohydrates for athletes.

2.1.2 Carbohydrate Recommendations for Athletes

Carbohydrate needs for athletes vary depending on the individual's size, sport, and training regimen. In general, the American College of Sports Medicine (ACSM) suggests that athletes consume 50-70% of their total daily calories from carbohydrates, with endurance athletes consuming the higher end of this range.

For optimal performance, the International Olympic Committee (IOC) recommends the following intake guidelines based on daily exercise volume:

- **Low-intensity exercise** (60 minutes or less) - 3-5 grams per kilogram of body weight
- **Moderate-intensity exercise** (60-120 minutes) - 5-7 grams per kilogram of body weight
- **High-intensity, prolonged exercise** (2.5-5 hours) - 8-10 grams per kilogram of body weight

Athletes should aim to consume complex carbohydrates throughout the day but simple carbohydrates during and immediately after exercise when rapid energy replenishment is necessary.

2.2 Proteins: Building Blocks for Athletes

Protein plays a significant role in the body, contributing to growth, repair, and maintenance of muscle tissue, as well as hormone production and immune function. For athletes, protein intake is crucial to support muscle recovery and adaptation after exercise.

2.2.1 Protein Sources

High-quality protein sources contain all essential amino acids (EAAs), which are the building blocks of proteins that the body cannot produce on its own. Some protein-rich foods include:

- Lean meats and poultry
- Fish and seafood
- Eggs and dairy products
- Soy and tofu
- Legumes, nuts, and seeds

2.2.2 Protein Recommendations for Athletes

The ACSM recommends that athletes consume 1.2-2.0 grams of protein per kilogram of body weight daily, with individuals participating in strength and power sports generally requiring protein at the higher end of this range. In addition, protein should be evenly distributed across meals and snacks, with athletes aiming for an intake of 20-30 grams per meal or snack.

2.3 Fats: Essential Energy Source and Nutrient Absorption

Fats serve many functions in the body, including energy production, insulation, and nutrient absorption. For athletes, fat intake is vital for optimal performance and recovery.

2.3.1 Types of Fats

There are three main types of fats:

- **Saturated Fats** - Typically found in animal-based products (e.g., fatty cuts of meat, butter, and full-fat dairy), saturated fats can be detrimental to cardiovascular health when consumed in excess. However, they serve essential functions in the body in moderation.
- **Unsaturated Fats** - Typically found in plant-based oils, nuts, seeds, and fatty fish, unsaturated fats are considered beneficial for cardiovascular health, with omega-3 fatty acids (found in fatty fish like salmon) crucial for reducing inflammation and supporting cognitive function.
- **Trans Fats** - Found in small amounts in some animal-based products and artificially in some processed foods, trans fats have been linked to an increased risk of cardiovascular disease and are best avoided by athletes.

2.3.2 Fat Recommendations for Athletes

The ACSM recommends that athletes consume 20-35% of their total daily calorie intake from fats, mainly focusing on healthy unsaturated fats. It's essential to avoid extreme fat restriction, as adequate fat intake supports hormone production, immune function, and vitamin absorption.

In summary, understanding the role of macronutrients—carbohydrates, proteins, and fats—is crucial for athletes in maximizing performance, supporting recovery, and ensuring overall health. Proper macronutrient intake should be tailored to each athlete's unique needs, depending on their sport, training, and goals.

Reference:

- "Nutrition and Athletic Performance." Medicine & Science in Sports & Exercise, vol. 48, no. 3, 2016, pp. 543-568, DOI: 10.1249/MSS.0000000000000852
- "Recommended Daily Macronutrient Intakes for Athletes", Australian Institute of Sport.

2.1 Carbohydrates: The Primary Energy Source

Carbohydrates are the body's preferred source of fuel during physical activity, providing energy for both high-intensity and lower-intensity exercises. Broadly speaking, carbohydrates can be classified into two categories: simple carbohydrates (also known as sugars) and complex carbohydrates (also referred to as starches or fibers). Understanding the breakdown and utilization of these types of carbs is essential for athletes looking to optimize their performance.

2.1.1 Simple Carbohydrates

Simple carbohydrates are composed of one or two sugar molecules, such as glucose, fructose, and sucrose, which provide a quick source of energy. Our body requires glucose to function, and the brain relies solely on glucose for energy. When consumed, simple carbohydrates result in a rapid increase in blood sugar levels, which can temporarily boost energy. Simple carbohydrates can be found in various food sources, such as fruits, milk, candies, and sports drinks.

For athletes, simple carbohydrates can be beneficial for short-duration, high-intensity activities as they provide quick energy to the muscles. During prolonged exercise, simple carbohydrates can also help maintain blood sugar levels, which can prevent fatigue and support continued performance.

However, despite their potential benefits, the regular consumption of large amounts of simple carbohydrates can lead to an increased risk of type 2 diabetes, obesity, and other health problems. Therefore, it is crucial for athletes to balance their simple carbohydrate intake with complex carbohydrates and other nutrients to maintain overall health.

2.1.2 Complex Carbohydrates

Unlike simple carbohydrates, complex carbohydrates are made of long chains of sugar molecules, such as starches and fibers. Due to their molecular structure, complex carbohydrates are broken down more slowly in the body, providing a steadier release of energy during activities. This slow digestion makes them ideal for maintaining consistent energy levels during endurance events, long training sessions, or any activity lasting longer than an hour.

Complex carbohydrates can be found in a variety of food sources, including whole grains, vegetables, legumes, and some fruits. These foods are not only higher in energy but also rich in essential vitamins, minerals, and fibers, which help maintain the proper function of the digestive system and promote overall health.

For athletes, incorporating complex carbohydrates into their diet is essential to supporting sustained energy levels for both training and competition. Research has shown that consuming complex carbohydrates before an event or training session can significantly enhance aerobic endurance and minimize feelings of fatigue. Moreover, replenishing carbohydrate stores by consuming complex carbohydrates within 30 minutes to an hour following exercise can aid in the recovery process and help prepare for the next workout.

2.1.3 Glycogen Storage and Importance

Carbohydrates are broken down into glucose and stored in the liver and muscles as glycogen. Glycogen is the body's primary fuel source during physical activity. However, our glycogen storage capacity is limited; once these stores are depleted during exercise, the body begins to break down fats and proteins to maintain energy production, which can eventually result in fatigue and reduced performance.

To ensure optimal glycogen storage, athletes should aim to consume adequate amounts of carbohydrates daily, as the body can store only a limited amount of carbohydrates as glycogen. Consuming adequate carbohydrates enables an athlete to maintain higher training intensities for longer durations, reducing the risk of fatigue.

2.1.4 Carbohydrate Intake Recommendations

The amount of carbohydrates an athlete should consume depends on their daily training volume, intensity, and individual nutritional needs. As a general guideline, the American Dietetic Association, Dietitians of Canada, and the

American College of Sports Medicine recommend the following carbohydrate intake for athletes:

- Low-intensity exercise (up to 1 hour per day): 3-5 grams of carbohydrates per kilogram of body weight per day
- Moderate-intensity exercise (1-3 hours per day): 5-7 grams of carbohydrates per kilogram of body weight per day
- High-intensity exercise (3-5 hours per day): 7-10 grams of carbohydrates per kilogram of body weight per day

In conclusion, carbohydrates are essential for athletes looking to optimize their performance. By understanding the different types of carbohydrates and their roles in energy production, athletes can better tailor their nutritional intake to support their daily activities and fuel their bodies for success.

2.1 Carbohydrates: The Energizer

Carbohydrates are often heralded as the primary fuel source for athletes. They can be broken down into two main categories: simple and complex carbohydrates. Simple carbohydrates are easily digestible and offer a rapid source of energy, while complex carbohydrates provide a sustained release of energy due to their slower digestive rate. Each type presents crucial benefits for athletic performance.

2.1.1 Simple Carbohydrates

Simple carbohydrates, also known as sugars, provide the body with instant energy. Upon consumption, they are rapidly absorbed into the bloodstream and supply an instant fuel resource for working muscles. Simple carbs can be further classified into two subcategories: monosaccharides and disaccharides.

Monosaccharides are the simplest form of carbohydrates and consist of a single sugar molecule. Examples include:

- Glucose: Also known as blood sugar, it is the primary source of energy for cells and is crucial for high-intensity exercise.
- Fructose: Found in many fruits, honey, and some vegetables.
- Galactose: A component of the lactose found in milk.

Disaccharides are formed by combining two monosaccharides. Well-known examples include:

- Sucrose (glucose + fructose): Commonly referred to as table sugar, it is made up of glucose and fructose.
- Lactose (glucose + galactose): The sugar found in milk and dairy products.
- Maltose (glucose + glucose): Found in malted grains and starches, it is a primary product of carbohydrate digestion.

Simple carbohydrates, while providing quick energy, can cause fluctuations in blood sugar levels, which may lead to short-term energy crashes. Therefore, consuming simple carbs should be strategically timed to ensure optimal performance during athletic events.

2.1.2 Complex Carbohydrates

Complex carbohydrates or polysaccharides, are composed of long chains of glucose molecules, which provide a steady, slow-release energy source. This makes them an essential component of an athlete's diet for maintaining energy levels during prolonged periods of exercise. There are two main types of complex carbohydrates: starches and dietary fiber.

Starches are the primary source of energy for humans, and their digestion begins in the mouth. They include two types of glucose chains: amylose and amylopectin. Starchy foods include:

- Whole grains such as wheat, oats, barley, and brown rice
- Legumes like beans, lentils, and peas
- Starchy vegetables like potatoes, corn, and pumpkin

Dietary fiber is a type of carbohydrate that cannot be fully broken down by digestive enzymes. There are two types of fiber: soluble and insoluble.

- Soluble fiber: It dissolves in water, forming a gel-like substance that helps slow down the absorption of nutrients, providing a feeling of fullness and stabilizing blood sugar levels. It can be found in oatmeal, nuts, seeds, legumes, and some fruits and vegetables.
- Insoluble fiber: It does not dissolve in water and aids in digestion by providing bulk to stool and promoting regular bowel movements. It can be found in whole grains, wheat bran, and numerous fruits and vegetables.

2.1.3 Carbohydrate Recommendations for Athletes

Carbohydrate consumption is highly individualized and varies depending on the type, intensity, and duration of an athlete's training regime. Generally, an athlete's carbohydrate intake should range between 45-65% of their total daily caloric intake. However, endurance athletes and those participating in high-intensity sports may require higher amounts to meet their energy demands.

Carbohydrate loading is a common practice utilized by endurance athletes, such as marathon runners, to maximize their glycogen stores before a race. This is done by increasing carbohydrate intake while reducing training intensity for several days preceding the event.

Additionally, consuming simple carbohydrates during an athletic event, such as a sports drink or energy gel, can help maintain energy levels and delay the onset of fatigue. Simple carbs can also be consumed immediately after an event to help replenish muscle glycogen stores and expedite recovery.

2.2 Proteins: Building Blocks for Success

Proteins are the foundation of various physiological processes, including tissue repair and regeneration, hormonal production, and enzyme synthesis. For athletes, protein is vital for the growth, repair, and maintenance of muscle tissue. It is composed of amino acids, which are often referred to as the "building blocks" of protein.

There are 20 amino acids in total, of which nine are classified as essential since they cannot be synthesized by the body and must be obtained through dietary sources. High-quality protein sources typically contain all the essential amino acids, which are crucial for optimal muscle recovery and development.

Common sources of high-quality protein include:

- Animal-derived products like meat, poultry, fish, eggs, and dairy
- Plant-based protein sources such as soy, quinoa, and legumes

2.2.1 Protein Requirements for Athletes

Protein needs vary depending on an athlete's type of sport, training intensity, and individual factors like age, weight, and body composition. Although the Recommended Daily Allowance (RDA) for protein is 0.8 grams per kilogram (g/kg) of body weight per day for the general population, athletes' requirements tend to be higher.

Current guidelines suggest that endurance athletes require 1.2-1.4 g/kg of body weight per day, while strength and power athletes may require 1.6-2.0 g/kg of body weight per day. Timing protein intake may also be key for maximizing muscle recovery and performance. Consuming a balanced meal containing protein within 0-2 hours post-exercise can promote muscle repair and rebuilding.

2.3 Fats: Fueling the Flames

Fats, or lipids, are essential for numerous processes within the body, such as hormone production, cell function, and the absorption of fat-soluble vitamins (A, D, E, K). They also provide a vital energy source, particularly for low to moderate intensity exercise when carbohydrate stores become depleted.

There are several types of dietary fats:

- Saturated fats: Typically found in animal products like beef, pork, and dairy; also found in some plant oils like coconut and palm oil
- Monounsaturated fats: Found in olive oil, avocados, and various nuts and seeds
- Polyunsaturated fats: Found in fatty fish, flaxseed, and some plant oils
- Trans fats: Found in some processed foods, such as margarine and commercially baked goods

Of these types of fat, monounsaturated and polyunsaturated fats are considered the most beneficial for health due to their potential to decrease inflammation and lower harmful cholesterol levels. Athletes should focus on incorporating these healthy fats into their diets while minimizing saturated and trans fat consumption.

2.3.1 Fat Requirements for Athletes

Fat requirements for athletes differ depending on factors such as body composition, type of sport, and individual goals. However, it is generally recommended that fat intake should comprise 20-35% of an athlete's total daily caloric intake. Although fat is a vital energy source, too much can lead to excess body fat and hinder athletic performance.

To optimize fat intake as an energy source for endurance exercise, athletes may practice "fat adaptation," which involves consuming more fat and fewer carbohydrates in the weeks leading up to an event. This may help lower the body's reliance on glycogen stores and improve overall performance.

In summary, carbohydrates, proteins, and fats each play crucial roles in meeting the energy, repair, and maintenance demands of athletes. Adequate intake of these macronutrients can lead to improved performance, faster recovery, and a lower risk of injury.

3. The Power of Micronutrients: Vitamins and Minerals for Athletes

3.1 Essential Vitamins: The Spark Plugs of Your Body

Vitamins are essential organic compounds that our bodies need for normal growth, development, and overall health. Unlike macronutrients (carbohydrates, fats, and proteins), vitamins are required in smaller amounts but are no less important. Acting as catalysts for various reactions and bodily functions, these micronutrients play a vital role in optimal bodily performance, particularly for athletes.

There are two main types of vitamins: fat-soluble and water-soluble. Fat-soluble vitamins, which include vitamins A, D, E, and K, are stored within the fatty tissues and liver for future use. Water-soluble vitamins, including B-complex vitamins and vitamin C, are not stored in the body and must be consumed regularly to maintain adequate levels.

3.1.1 Roles of Vitamins in Athletic Performance

Vitamins play many roles in maintaining overall health and supporting athletic performance, including:

- *Energy production*: B-complex vitamins like thiamin (B1), riboflavin (B2), and niacin (B3) play a significant role in converting nutrients into energy during exercise. For athletes, proper intake of these B vitamins allows their bodies to more efficiently metabolize and utilize macronutrients for fuel, which translates to more effective workouts and recovery.

- *Antioxidant defense*: Vitamins C and E act as powerful antioxidants that protect cells from free radicals generated during exercise. Ensuring adequate intake of these antioxidants helps athletes manage oxidative stress, which can lead to inflammation and muscle damage, thus enhancing recovery and reducing the risk of injury.
- *Bone health*: Vitamin D helps your body absorb and use calcium and phosphorous to maintain strong bones and teeth. As athletes are more prone to bone-related injuries, maintaining adequate vitamin D levels is crucial.
- *Immune function*: Intense physical activity can temporarily suppress the immune system, which can increase susceptibility to illness and infection. Vitamins C and B6 play key roles in supporting the immune system, which is especially important for athletes during high-intensity training periods.
- *Muscle repair and growth*: Vitamin A is involved in the synthesis of proteins, which are essential for muscle repair and growth. Adequate vitamin A intake is crucial for athletes looking to build muscle and recover effectively from workouts.

3.1.2 Dietary Sources of Vitamins

To ensure adequate consumption of vitamins, athletes should aim to consume a variety of foods from all food groups. Some examples of good dietary sources of vitamins include:

- *B-complex vitamins*: These vitamins can be found in a wide range of foods, including whole grains, lean meats, poultry, fish, eggs, dairy products, nuts, seeds, and leafy green vegetables.
- *Vitamin C*: This antioxidant vitamin can be found in abundance in citrus fruits, red and green peppers, kiwifruit, strawberries, broccoli, and spinach.
- *Vitamin E*: Rich sources of this fat-soluble vitamin include nuts, seeds, vegetable oils, whole grains, and leafy green vegetables.
- *Vitamin A*: This vitamin is found in both animal and plant-based foods. Good sources include liver, fish, dairy products, carrots, sweet potatoes, spinach, and kale.
- *Vitamin D*: The best natural sources of vitamin D are fatty fish like salmon, mackerel, and sardines. Fortified milk and milk derivatives, like cheese and yogurt, are also good sources of this vitamin. In addition, modest exposure to sunlight can help your body produce vitamin D.

3.1.3 Ensuring Adequate Vitamin Intake

While it's crucial for athletes to ensure adequate vitamin intake, consuming excessive amounts can lead to toxicity or create imbalances with other nutrients. To maintain optimal health and performance, it's essential to:

1. *Focus on nutrient-dense foods*: Consuming a variety of fruits, vegetables, whole grains, lean proteins, and healthy fats can provide the majority of athletes' vitamin needs. Strive for a colorful plate, as vibrant fruits and vegetables tend to be packed with essential nutrients.
2. *Be mindful of supplementation*: Athletes should consult a healthcare professional or sports nutritionist

before using vitamin supplements, to assess potential deficiencies or imbalances. In cases where an individual is unable to meet their vitamin needs through regular diet, supplementation may be advised.

3. *Monitor vitamin status*: Regularly assessing blood nutrient levels can help identify potential deficiencies or imbalances, and provide helpful information to guide dietary changes or supplementation.

By understanding the significant roles vitamins play in athletic performance, athletes can optimize their diet to ensure they're consuming adequate amounts of these essential micronutrients. Doing so will not only support overall health but will also contribute to a more efficient and effective approach to training and recovery.

3.1 Importance of Micronutrients for Athletic Performance

Micronutrients, comprising mainly of vitamins and minerals, are essential to overall health, proper functioning of the body, and athletic performance. Although needed in small quantities compared to macronutrients (proteins, fats, and carbohydrates), micronutrients play crucial roles in energy production, tissue repair, and immune function - all vital aspects for athletes.

3.1.1 Vitamins for Athletes

Vitamins are organic compounds that the body needs in order to grow and develop normally. Two groups of vitamins are crucial for athletes: water-soluble and fat-soluble vitamins. The water-soluble vitamins (vitamin C and B-complex vitamins) are easily absorbed by the body, while the fat-soluble vitamins (vitamins A, D, E, and K) dissolve in fats and can be stored in the body for longer periods.

- **Vitamin C** - Also known as ascorbic acid, vitamin C plays a significant role in collagen synthesis, which is important for healthy bones, skin, and connective tissues. It also functions as a powerful antioxidant, supports the immune system, and aids in iron absorption. You can find abundant vitamin C in citrus fruits, strawberries, spinach, and potatoes.
- **B-complex Vitamins** - The B-complex vitamins include B1 (thiamine), B2 (riboflavin), B3 (niacin), B5 (pantothenic acid), B6 (pyridoxine), B7 (biotin), B9 (folic acid), and B12 (cobalamin). These vitamins play a significant role in energy metabolism, red blood cell production, nerve function, and the body's repair processes. Good sources of B vitamins include whole grains, legumes, seeds, and a variety of fruits and vegetables.
- **Vitamin A** - Vital for vision, growth, and immune function, vitamin A also contributes to tissue repair, making it essential for athletes. Vitamin A is found in foods like liver, sweet potatoes, carrots, spinach, and apricots.
- **Vitamin D** - Important for its role in calcium absorption, vitamin D is key for bone health and the prevention of stress fractures in athletes. The body can produce vitamin D when the skin is exposed to sunlight. It can also be found in foods such as fatty fish, egg yolks, and fortified milk.
- **Vitamin E** - Known for its antioxidant properties, vitamin E helps protect cells from damage by neutralizing free radicals, which are generated during workouts. You can find vitamin E in nuts, seeds, and vegetable oils.

- **Vitamin K** - Essential for blood clotting and bone metabolism, vitamin K plays a role in preventing injuries and maintaining strong bones in athletes. Foods rich in vitamin K include leafy greens, broccoli, and brussels sprouts.

3.1.2 Minerals for Athletes

Minerals are inorganic substances that are important for various functions in the body, such as maintaining fluid balance, nerve transmission, and muscle contraction. Some key minerals for athletes are:

- **Calcium** - Critical for bone health and muscle function, calcium is an essential mineral for athletes to prevent weak bones and muscle cramps. Dairy products, leafy greens, and fortified foods are rich sources of calcium.
- **Iron** - An important component of hemoglobin in red blood cells, iron helps transport oxygen throughout the body. Low iron levels can lead to anemia, which can impair athletic performance. Athletes, especially female and endurance athletes, need to ensure they consume adequate iron through foods like lean meat, poultry, fish, beans, and fortified cereals.
- **Magnesium** - Crucial for over 300 biochemical reactions in the body, magnesium maintains nerve and muscle function, supports the immune system, and aids in energy production. Athletes can find magnesium in nuts, seeds, whole grains, and green leafy vegetables.
- **Potassium** - A key electrolyte, potassium assists with nerve transmission, muscle contraction, and fluid balance. It is especially important for athletes who lose potassium through sweat during exercise.

Potassium-rich foods include bananas, potatoes, spinach, and yogurt.
- **Sodium** - Another essential electrolyte, sodium plays a vital role in fluid balance and nerve transmission. Athletes lose sodium through sweat and need to replenish it, especially during prolonged or intense exercise. Sodium can be found in table salt, sports drinks, and many processed foods.

In conclusion, micronutrients play a significant role in maintaining optimal athletic performance by supporting various functions in the body. A well-rounded diet that includes a wide variety of colorful fruits and vegetables, whole grains, lean proteins, and healthy fats should provide most of the essential vitamins and minerals needed by athletes. In some cases, supplementation may be necessary after consultation with a healthcare professional or registered dietitian.

3.1 The Importance of Micronutrients in Athletic Performance

While macronutrients, such as carbohydrates, proteins, and fats, are often at the forefront of an athlete's nutrition plan, micronutrients also play a crucial role in optimizing athletic performance. Micronutrients, consisting of vitamins and minerals, are required in smaller amounts than macronutrients, yet they're essential for overall health, proper functioning of the body, and ultimately, peak performance in sports.

Micronutrients should not be overlooked in the diet of athletes, as they participate in various physiological processes such as energy production, muscle function, red blood cell formation, and immune system support. Adequate consumption of vitamins and minerals through a well-balanced diet ensures that an athlete's body operates efficiently, recovers well, and adapts to the demands of training and competition.

3.1.1 Vitamins: The Catalysts of Bodily Functions

Vitamins are organic compounds required in small amounts to support the proper functioning of the body. They act as catalysts in various chemical reactions, ensuring that essential processes occur at optimal rates. There are two categories of vitamins: fat-soluble and water-soluble.

Fat-Soluble Vitamins include vitamins A, D, E, and K, which are stored in the body's fat tissue and therefore not required daily. They play essential roles in:

- Vision (Vitamin A)
- Bone health and calcium regulation (Vitamin D)
- Antioxidant activity (Vitamin E)
- Blood clotting (Vitamin K)

Water-Soluble Vitamins include the B complex vitamins (B1, B2, B3, B5, B6, B7, B9, B12) and vitamin C, which are not stored in the body and must be regularly replenished through diet. They play essential roles in:

- Energy production (B vitamins)
- Red blood cell formation (Vitamins B9 and B12)
- Antioxidant activity and collagen synthesis (Vitamin C)

Athletes should ensure they consume adequate amounts of both fat-soluble and water-soluble vitamins throughout their training period, as deficiencies in specific vitamins can lead to various health issues and impaired athletic performance.

3.1.2 Minerals: The Building Blocks of Athletic Performance

Minerals, inorganic substances required in small amounts, are crucial for different bodily functions. Some common minerals that athletes must pay attention to include calcium, magnesium, iron, and sodium.

Calcium is a major component of bones and teeth, playing a crucial role in skeletal strength and development. It also aids in muscle contractions, nerve transmission, and blood coagulation. Athletes, particularly those who participate in high-impact sports, must ensure they consume enough calcium to maintain bone health and reduce the risk of fractures.

Magnesium is involved in over 300 enzyme systems in the body, supporting muscle and nerve function, regulating blood pressure, and assisting with energy production. A deficiency in magnesium can lead to muscle cramps, fatigue, and compromised cardiovascular function, hindering athletic performance.

Iron is vital for transporting oxygen to cells through hemoglobin and myoglobin proteins, and it contributes to energy production as a component of various enzymatic reactions. In athletes, iron deficiency can reduce aerobic capacity, lower endurance, and impair overall performance. Enhanced iron requirements are common in endurance athletes due to increased red blood cell production in response to the demands of training.

Sodium is a primary electrolyte that helps regulate fluid balance, muscle contractions, and nerve function. Athletes who engage in vigorous exercise, especially in hot environments, must ensure they consume enough sodium to replace losses through sweat and maintain proper hydration.

Athletes should aim to consume a balanced diet rich in nutrient-dense foods to meet mineral requirements, as inadequacies can pose risks to performance, recovery, and injury prevention.

3.1.3 Micronutrient Timing and Sources

The timing of micronutrient intake is less critical than macronutrient timing; however, consuming essential vitamins and minerals consistently is crucial for athletes. To ensure adequate intake, athletes should aim to consume a varied diet composed of whole, unprocessed foods in balanced meals and snacks throughout the day.

To maximize their micronutrient intake, athletes should include a variety of colorful fruits and vegetables, dairy products, whole grains, lean proteins, nuts, seeds, and fortified foods in their diets.

In some cases, athletes may require supplementation to meet their micronutrient needs, especially if they have specific dietary restrictions or deficiencies. However, supplementation should be approached with caution, as excessive intake of certain micronutrients can negatively impact health. It is crucial to consult with a healthcare practitioner or sports dietitian before beginning any supplementation regimen.

3.1.4 Conclusion

Micronutrients are essential for overall health and play a significant role in the performance and recovery of athletes. By consuming a balanced and varied diet, athletes can ensure they receive the necessary vitamins and minerals to optimize their training and achieve peak performance.

4. Hydration Strategies and Electrolytes: Staying Ahead of Dehydration

4.1 Understanding the Importance of Hydration in Sports Performance

Before diving into various hydration strategies, it is crucial to understand why proper hydration is crucial for optimal sports performance. Water is a central component in the human body, making up around 60% of the body composition. It plays numerous essential roles such as maintaining blood volume, regulating body temperature, transporting nutrients, and removing waste products from our body. Thus, even slight shifts in the body's hydration status can have profound effects on an athlete's performance, recovery, and risk of injury.

4.1.1 Dehydration and its Impact on Performance

Dehydration occurs when water loss exceeds water intake, leading to a decrease in the body's water content. This can happen through sweating, respiration, and urination, all of which are accelerated during periods of intense exercise. Dehydration can have significant consequences for athletic performance, some of which include:

- **Reduced endurance:** Dehydration results in reduced blood volume, leading to decreased oxygen transportation to muscles and increased heart rate.

This increased cardiovascular strain can contribute to reduced endurance and a decline in performance.

- **Impaired thermoregulation:** Proper hydration is essential for maintaining body temperature during exercise. When dehydrated, an athlete's sweating response is reduced, and more heat is stored, consequently increasing the risk of heat illnesses such as heat cramps, heat exhaustion, and heatstroke.
- **Increased perceived exertion:** Dehydration can affect an athlete's mental and physical perception of exercise intensity, making exercise feel more challenging than it should. This increased perceived exertion can lead to premature fatigue and a decline in performance.
- **Decreased mental function:** Cognitive function, such as decision-making, attention, and memory, can also be impaired due to dehydration. In sports that require quick decisions, precision, and coordination, the impact of dehydration on mental function may be detrimental to performance.

4.1.2 The Role of Electrolytes in Staying Hydrated

Electrolytes, such as sodium, potassium, calcium, and magnesium, play a vital role in maintaining a proper hydration balance. They are charged particles that help regulate fluid balance, muscle contractions, and nerve function. During periods of intense exercise, athletes lose electrolytes through sweat, predominantly sodium and potassium. To maintain optimal sports performance, it is essential to replenish these lost electrolytes. Thus, sports drinks that contain electrolytes are often recommended for athletes, especially during prolonged or intense training sessions.

4.2 Practical Hydration Strategies for Athletes

Proper hydration involves more than just drinking plenty of fluids. Athletes need to develop a personalized hydration plan to account for individual sweat rates, electrolyte losses, and fluid preferences. The following strategies may help athletes stay ahead of dehydration:

4.2.1 Pre-hydration

To start exercise or competition in a properly hydrated state, follow these guidelines:

- Ensure adequate daily fluid intake by consuming at least 2-3 liters of water or other fluids per day, depending on the individual needs and physical activity levels.
- Monitor urine color: Aim for a light yellow color as an indicator of proper hydration.
- Consume a pre-exercise meal or snack containing sodium and fluids about 2-3 hours before exercise to help stimulate thirst and retain consumed fluids.

4.2.2 Hydration During Exercise

Keeping a close eye on hydration during exercise can help prevent dehydration and maintain sports performance. Consider these strategies for maintaining hydration during exercise:

- Monitor individual sweat rate by weighing yourself before and after exercise, adjusting for fluid intake

during exercise. Aim to replace fluid losses as close to your sweat rate as possible without overhydrating.
- Consume fluids at regular intervals throughout exercise (every 10-20 minutes) to maintain hydration, even if you don't feel thirsty.
- Choose sports drinks containing electrolytes, especially sodium and potassium, to replace electrolyte losses due to sweating. This is particularly important during prolonged or intense exercise, or when competing in hot environments.

4.2.3 Rehydration

After exercise, prioritize rehydration to aid in recovery and prepare for the next training session or competition. Some effective rehydration strategies include:

- Within the first 30-60 minutes post-exercise, consume a sports drink or other electrolyte-rich fluids to replace sweat losses and lost electrolytes.
- Continue rehydrating with additional fluids in the hours following exercise, aiming to consume 1.25-1.5 liters of fluid per kilogram of body weight lost.
- Ensure a sodium-rich meal or snack is consumed post-exercise to help retain fluids and replace lost electrolytes.

By understanding the importance of hydration and implementing practical strategies to stay ahead of dehydration, athletes can optimize their sports performance, reduce the risk of injury, and ensure a faster recovery. As every individual is unique, taking a personalized approach to hydration and monitoring individual sweat rates is essential for maximizing performance and health.

4.1 Importance of Hydration

Adequate hydration is crucial for athletes for optimizing performance and ensuring overall health. Water is involved in many metabolic processes and physiological adaptations, such as regulating body temperature, transporting nutrients, and maintaining blood volume. Furthermore, water is indispensable for joint lubrication and protecting sensitive tissues.

During athletic events, the body loses fluids through sweat, respiration, and other processes, leading to dehydration if not adequately replenished. Dehydration can severely affect an athlete's performance, causing fatigue, impaired cognition, reduced endurance, and increased risk of heat-related illnesses. Therefore, it is essential to maintain an effective hydration strategy throughout training and competition.

4.2 Fluid Balance and Dehydration

Fluid balance refers to the equilibrium between water intake and water losses. An athlete's body achieves fluid balance when the amount of fluids consumed equals the amount of fluids expended. Any discrepancy in fluid balance can result in dehydration, leading to various symptoms and reduced performance.

Signs of dehydration include:

- Thirst
- Dry mouth and throat
- Dark-colored urine
- Decreased urine output
- Rapid heartbeat
- Lightheadedness
- Muscle cramps

To assess one's hydration status, athletes should monitor their urine color and frequency. Ideally, urine should be light yellow and in regular frequency.

4.3 Individualized Hydration Strategy

Athletes should establish an individualized hydration strategy to meet their unique fluid needs. Factors affecting an athlete's fluid requirements include:

- Duration and intensity of exercise
- Environmental conditions (temperature or altitude)
- Sweat rate
- Acclimatization to the environment
- Genetic predisposition for sweating
- Body size and composition

To develop an effective hydration strategy, athletes should do the following:

1. Assess their sweat rate by weighing themselves pre- and post-workout, with exercise sessions lasting at least an hour. Since each kilogram of body weight lost represents approximately 1-liter water loss, this measure can help athletes estimate how much fluid they need to drink to replenish lost fluids.
2. Learn their individual fluid preferences considering taste, texture, temperature, and type. This can help optimize fluid intake during training and competition.
3. Practice timed drinking strategies, such as drinking small amounts of fluids every 15-20 minutes during exercise, to help maintain fluid balance throughout.
4. Pre-hydrate about 2-3 hours before exercise by consuming 0.5 to 1 liter of fluids. This can optimize physiologic function and improve exercise performance.

5. Pay attention to post-exercise hydration as well to replenish lost fluids, particularly during multi-day events or training sessions.

4.4 Electrolytes

Electrolytes are essential minerals dissolved in blood and other bodily fluids, playing a significant role in many physiological processes. The primary electrolytes include sodium, potassium, chloride, calcium, and magnesium. These electrolytes regulate fluid balance, muscle contraction, nerve function, and pH balance.

During athletic events, the body loses not only water but also electrolytes through sweat. Replacing lost electrolytes is crucial for maintaining optimal performance and preventing adverse health outcomes. Without proper electrolyte balance, an athlete may experience muscle cramping, fatigue, weakness, irregular heartbeat, or even severe health risks like hyponatremia.

To maintain electrolyte balance, athletes should consider consuming sports drinks containing electrolytes during prolonged exercise or in hot and humid conditions. Alternatively, electrolyte tablets or powders can be added to water for a customizable electrolyte source. Athletes should also maintain a balanced and nutrient-dense diet to ensure they obtain essential electrolytes from their daily meals.

4.5 Practical Tips for Hydration Management

- Always have fluids readily available during training and competition.
- Begin exercise well-hydrated by consuming 0.5 to 1 liter of fluids 2-3 hours before the activity.

- Choose a fluid source that is palatable to promote consistent consumption during exercise.
- Include electrolytes in your hydration strategy during prolonged exercise or in hot and humid conditions.
- Monitor your hydration status by tracking urine color and frequency.
- Remember that individual needs vary; regularly assess and adjust your hydration strategy accordingly.

In conclusion, incorporating proper hydration strategies, including adequate water intake and electrolyte replenishment, can significantly improve an athlete's performance, recovery, and health. Each athlete should create an individualized hydration plan based on their unique fluid requirements and preferences, and continually evaluate and adjust the plan as needed. By staying ahead of dehydration, athletes can set themselves up for optimal success in training and competition.

4.1 Understanding Dehydration and Its Effect on Performance

Dehydration occurs when an athlete loses more fluids, primarily through sweating and respiration, than they take in during exercise. As an athlete, it's important to understand that even mild dehydration can adversely affect physical and mental performance, leading to a reduction in endurance, strength, and decision-making abilities. Moreover, dehydration can have longer-term effects on overall health, making it essential to prioritize proper hydration strategies.

Dehydration: The Science Behind It

Our bodies are made up of approximately 60% water, which plays a critical role in maintaining proper cellular function, regulating body temperature, and helping transport nutrients in and out of cells. During exercise, the body's core temperature rises, and the body cools down by producing sweat. As sweat evaporates from the skin, this helps to dissipate heat and maintain a safe body temperature.

However, the water loss through sweat can lead to dehydration if fluids are not replenished properly, resulting in decreased blood volume, increased heart rate, and reduced ability to supply muscles with oxygen, ultimately leading to impaired performance.

How Hydration Affects Athletic Performance

1. **Endurance:** Dehydration can lead to reduced cardiovascular efficiency, as blood volume decreases and the body has to work harder to pump oxygen and nutrients to the muscles. Even a 2% reduction in body weight due to fluid loss can lead to a decline in endurance, so hydration is essential in maintaining peak performance during endurance events.
2. **Strength and power:** Both muscle strength and power can be compromised when the body is dehydrated. Cellular function within the muscle becomes less efficient with reduced fluid availability, leading to decreased force production and overall strength.
3. **Cognitive function:** Dehydration can lead to impaired decision-making, reduced concentration, and diminished reaction time. In sports where quick thinking and strategy are crucial, maintaining proper hydration is key to maintaining mental clarity and focus.

4. **Thermoregulation:** As mentioned above, the body cools down through the process of sweating. If dehydration occurs, the body's ability to regulate temperature becomes compromised, leading to overheating and potentially dangerous consequences such as heatstroke.
5. **Recovery:** Adequate hydration is necessary for optimal recovery, as fluids are required for the transport of nutrients to muscles and the elimination of waste products. Inadequate hydration can lead to delayed recovery and increased muscle soreness.

Electrolytes: The Role They Play in Hydration

Electrolytes are minerals that help maintain the balance of fluids within the body and assists in various critical functions such as muscle contractions, nerve function, and pH balance. The most relevant electrolytes to athletes are sodium, potassium, calcium, and magnesium. During exercise, electrolytes are lost through sweat, and it's essential to replenish them to sustain athletic performance.

1. **Sodium:** The primary electrolyte lost in sweat, sodium helps to regulate fluid balance and maintain blood volume. Inadequate sodium intake can lead to muscle cramps, dizziness, and in severe cases, hyponatremia (low blood sodium levels).
2. **Potassium:** Working in tandem with sodium, potassium is another vital electrolyte required for proper muscle and nerve function. A deficiency can contribute to muscle cramps, weakness, and fatigue.
3. **Calcium:** Essential for proper nerve function, muscle contractions, and bone health, calcium is crucial for athletes. Along with other electrolytes, low calcium levels can contribute to muscle cramps and impaired performance.

4. **Magnesium:** Involved in hundreds of biochemical reactions within the body, magnesium plays a crucial role in energy production, nerve function, and muscle contractions. Low magnesium levels can lead to muscle cramps, weakness, and fatigue.

4.2 Developing Optimal Hydration Strategies for Athletes

Now that we understand the importance of hydration and electrolyte balance, it's time to discuss strategies to maintain optimal hydration before, during, and after exercise.

Pre-Exercise Hydration

To ensure proper hydration before exercise, athletes should drink between 16-20 ounces (~450-600 mL) of water or a sports drink containing electrolytes approximately two hours before the activity. This allows time for your body to absorb the fluid and regulate excess if necessary, helping you begin your exercise well-hydrated. Aiming for pale-yellow urine color is a useful indicator of adequate hydration.

Hydration During Exercise

During exercise, the amount of fluid and electrolyte requirements varies depending on factors like duration, intensity, and environmental conditions. As a general guideline, athletes should aim to drink 7-10 ounces (~200-300 mL) of hydrating fluid every 10-20 minutes. For workouts lasting longer than an hour or in hot and humid environments, consider using a sports drink containing electrolytes to replace those lost through sweat.

It's essential to avoid a "one size fits all" approach to hydration, as individual sweat rates can vary significantly. Monitoring your weight before and after exercise, and keeping track of any fluid intake during the activity, can help you better understand your unique fluid needs over time.

Post-Exercise Rehydration

After exercise, it's crucial to restore fluids and electrolytes in the body. Aim to drink at least 16-20 ounces (~450-600 mL) of water or a sports drink containing electrolytes for every pound (0.5 kg) of body weight lost during the activity. Don't rely solely on thirst to determine your fluid needs, as thirst can be an unreliable indicator, particularly after high-intensity exercise.

Proper hydration and electrolyte balance are key components to athletic success, and understanding individual fluid needs can make a significant difference in performance and overall health. By implementing the outlined strategies and monitoring fluid intake, athletes will be well-equipped to stay ahead of dehydration and reach their full potential.

4.1 The Science of Hydration and Dehydration

4.1.1 The Importance of Water in the Body

Water is essential for life and plays a critical role in the overall health and function of the body. It provides structure to cells, transports nutrients to organs and tissues, lubricates joints, and is involved in critical chemical reactions in the body. As athletes, hydration is especially important because it directly impacts physical and mental performance, as well as recovery.

During exercise, the body's demand for water and electrolytes dramatically increases as it works to regulate and maintain core temperature. Sweat is produced, and with it, important electrolytes like sodium and potassium are lost. If too much fluid is lost through sweat and not replaced, dehydration sets in, making it difficult for the body to effectively function and perform at optimal levels.

4.1.2 Dehydration and Athletic Performance

Dehydration can have a significant impact on an athlete's performance, strength, endurance, and recovery. Even a modest loss of 1-2% of body weight in fluids can contribute to reduced mental and physical performance. Some of the negative effects of dehydration on athletes include:

- Reduced blood volume, leading to an increased heart rate and perceived exertion.
- Decreased sweat production and increased core temperature, leading to a higher risk of heat-related illnesses.
- Impaired cognitive function, reaction time, and decision-making abilities.
- Decreased muscle strength and endurance.
- Increased risk of cramps due to electrolyte imbalances.
- Slower recovery from training and competition as dehydration can hinder the body's natural healing processes.

With these considerations in mind, it becomes clear that proper hydration is essential for optimal performance and recovery.

4.1.3 Assessing Hydration Status

To effectively implement hydration strategies, athletes should regularly monitor their hydration status. There are several methods to evaluate and track hydration levels, including:

1. **Urine color:** Light, pale-yellow urine generally indicates proper hydration, while dark yellow or amber-colored urine suggests dehydration.
2. **Weight changes:** Changes in body weight after training sessions can represent fluid losses. A reduction of 1-2% or greater indicates dehydration.
3. **Thirst:** If an athlete experiences thirst during or after training, it is an indicator that they need to drink. It's important to note that thirst occurs after the body is already experiencing mild dehydration.

4.1.4 Key Components of an Effective Hydration Strategy

1. **Pre-hydration:** Athletes should drink fluids regularly before exercise to maintain a state of hydration. This involves consuming 5-10 ml/kg body weight of water or sports drink at least 2-4 hours before exercise.
2. **During exercise:** Athletes should consume fluids regularly to match sweat loss, prevent dehydration, and maintain electrolyte balance. Generally, it is recommended to drink 7-10 ounces of fluid every 10-20 minutes during exercise. Adjust rates to match individual sweat rates and environmental conditions, as well as the intensity of exercise.
3. **Post-exercise:** For every pound of body weight lost due to sweat, athletes should aim to consume 20-24 ounces of fluid within 2 hours of exercise completion.

4. **Electrolyte replenishment:** Consuming sports drinks or electrolyte supplements aids in the replenishment of electrolytes like sodium and potassium lost through sweat. This can help prevent cramps, support muscle function, and maintain proper neural communication.
5. **Individualization:** Understand that hydration needs vary among individuals based on factors like sweat rate, body weight, and environmental conditions. Regularly tracking and assessing personal hydration needs will help determine the most effective hydration strategy for optimal performance and recovery.

By understanding the science of dehydration and the importance of hydration in the body, athletes can implement effective hydration strategies that cater to their unique needs, allowing them to maintain top-level physical and mental performance, minimize the risk of heat-related illnesses, and optimize recovery.

4.1 Why Hydration is Crucial for Athletes

Water is the most vital component of the human body, composing roughly 60% of body weight. Proper hydration is essential for various physiological processes, including temperature regulation, nutrient transportation, and waste elimination. For athletes, staying adequately hydrated has additional advantages like enhanced performance, reduced fatigue, and faster recovery.

4.1.1 The Role of Water in Athletic Performance

During exercise, the body sweats to cool down its core temperature, thereby losing water and essential electrolytes through sweat. If this fluid loss is not replaced, dehydration can set in and severely impair an athlete's performance, as demonstrated by these key effects:

1. **Reduced Endurance**: Dehydration decreases blood volume, which in turn lowers the amount of oxygen supplied to muscles, resulting in quicker fatigue.
2. **Poor Muscle Function**: Lack of water can cause muscles to cramp, reducing an athlete's ability to perform at their best.
3. **Decreased Coordination**: Dehydration can negatively impact an athlete's reaction time and cognitive functioning, ultimately hindering their overall performance.
4. **Increased Risk of Heat Illness**: Keeping your body temperature within a healthy range is facilitated by staying adequately hydrated, as water is essential for proper thermoregulation. Without sufficient hydration, the risk of heat-related illnesses, such as heat strokes or heat exhaustion, increases.

4.1.2 Hydration Strategies: Fluid Intake Recommendations

A customized hydration plan is crucial for athletes to perform optimally and stay adequately hydrated. The following guidelines can help athletes establish a proper hydration strategy:

- **Pre-exercise**: Ideally, athletes should drink 14 to 22 ounces (400 to 600 milliliters) of fluid within two hours before exercising to ensure they have adequate base hydration.
- **During exercise**: Athletes should aim to consume water or sports drinks at regular intervals throughout the workout, preferably every 10 to 20 minutes. A

basic guideline is to drink 7 to 10 ounces (200 to 300 milliliters) of fluid per 10 to 20 minutes of activity.
- **Post-exercise**: The goal here is to replenish any fluid losses incurred during exercise. Athletes can calculate their individualized fluid needs by weighing themselves before and after exercise. For every pound (0.5 kilograms) of lost body weight, consume 16 to 24 ounces (500 to 750 milliliters) of fluid.

4.1.3 Electrolytes: Balancing the Body's Needs

Electrolytes are essential minerals that conduct electrical impulses and maintain fluid balance in the body. Key electrolytes include sodium, potassium, calcium, and magnesium. During exercise, athletes lose electrolytes through sweat, potentially causing an imbalance that may lead to cramping, irregular heartbeat, or even more severe consequences.

For moderate-to-high intensity workouts lasting more than one hour, athletes should consider consuming an electrolyte-containing sports drink to replenish lost minerals. Most sports drinks contain sodium and potassium, while others also include calcium and magnesium.

Tips for Choosing the Right Sports Drink:

1. **Sodium Content**: Aim for a sports drink containing 50 to 165 milligrams of sodium per 8 ounces (240 milliliters). Sodium helps replace losses from sweat and encourages fluid retention.
2. **Potassium Content**: Choose a sports drink containing 20 to 50 milligrams of potassium per 8 ounces (240 milliliters). Potassium helps balance fluid levels and contributes to muscle function.

3. **Carbohydrates**: A sports drink should have a carbohydrate concentration of 6% to 8%. This level provides enough easily digestible carbohydrates to fuel workouts without causing stomach discomfort.
4. **Taste**: Finally, choose a sports drink with a taste you enjoy; this will encourage adequate consumption during exercise.

4.1.4 The Importance of Monitoring Hydration Levels

Monitoring your hydration status helps ensure that you are consuming enough fluids to optimize performance and prevent dehydration. Simple methods to track hydration levels include:

- **Urine color**: A well-hydrated athlete should produce clear or pale yellow urine. Dark yellow or amber-colored urine may indicate dehydration.
- **Thirst**: While thirst is a useful indicator of necessary fluid consumption, be sure to drink fluids consistently throughout your workout, as thirst may not be apparent until you are already dehydrated.
- **Sweat rate**: By calculating your sweat rate (i.e., the amount of sweat lost during exercise), you can better understand your individual fluid needs. Weigh yourself before and after exercise and replace each pound (0.5 kilograms) of lost weight with 16 to 24 ounces (500 to 750 milliliters) of fluid.

4.1.5 Hydration Strategies for Various Conditions

Factors such as the climate, altitude, and individual differences can impact an athlete's hydration needs. Be sure to adjust your fluid intake accordingly to maintain proper hydration:

- **Hot or humid conditions**: Higher temperatures and humidity lead to increased sweat rates. Adjust your fluid intake to account for these additional losses.
- **Cold conditions**: Athletes often underestimate their fluid needs in colder conditions. Be mindful of your hydration levels, as the body continues to lose fluids through respiration and sweating even in low temperatures.
- **High altitude**: At elevated altitudes, the body's fluid losses are accelerated due to increased respiratory rates and lower humidity levels. Stay adequately hydrated by increasing your fluid consumption.
- **Individual differences**: Factors such as body size, fitness level, and sweat rates can influence your fluid needs. Monitor your hydration status and adjust your fluid intake to suit your specific needs.

In the world of sports and fitness, remaining properly hydrated is critical for success. By implementing a tailored hydration strategy using the comprehensive information outlined above, athletes can maximize their performance, recovery, and overall well-being. Stay on top of your hydration, and watch your athleticism soar to new heights.

5. Pre-Workout Nutrition: Priming the Body for Optimal Performance

5.1 Importance of Pre-Workout Nutrition: Laying the Foundations for Success

The significance of pre-workout nutrition cannot be overstated as it plays a vital role in preparing the body for exercise and athletic performance by providing the necessary fuel to maximize energy levels, strength, and endurance. A well-thought-out pre-workout nutrition plan can reduce muscle breakdown, decrease the risk of injury, and enhance the overall performance during a workout. This section delves into the types of nutrients necessary for pre-workout nutrition, how they function, and the optimal timings to consume these nutrients.

5.1.1 Macronutrients for Pre-Workout Nutrition

The major macronutrients that contribute to an effective pre-workout nutrition plan are carbohydrates, proteins, and fats. Each of these components plays a unique and indispensable role in fueling the body for optimal performance during a workout session.

- **Carbohydrates**
  Carbohydrates serve as the primary source of energy for the body. Consuming carbohydrates before a workout can optimize glycogen stores, which

ultimately leads to better performance and endurance. There are two types of carbohydrates: simple and complex. Simple carbohydrates, such as fruits and sports drinks, are easily digestible and therefore provide a quick source of energy. Complex carbohydrates, like whole grains and high-fiber vegetables, take longer to digest and gradually release energy, helping to maintain energy levels throughout the exercise session.

For pre-workout nutrition, it is recommended to consume a combination of simple and complex carbohydrates to ensure both immediate and sustained energy release during the workout. The recommended consumption of carbohydrates is approximately 0.5 - 1g of carbohydrates per pound of body weight 3 - 4 hours before exercising.

- **Proteins**

Proteins are not primary sources of energy during exercise, but they play a crucial role in muscle repair and recovery. Consuming protein before a workout can reduce muscle breakdown and promote muscle growth. Including protein-rich sources like lean meats, dairy, or plant-based proteins in your pre-workout meal can provide the necessary amino acids to aid in muscle synthesis and recovery. Research suggests that 15 - 30g of protein within 3 - 4 hours before a workout is recommended for optimal performance.

- **Fats**

Fats are essential for providing energy, especially during aerobic exercises of duration longer than 1 hour. Fat digestion is relatively slow compared to carbohydrates and proteins, which acts as a benefit because fats can provide a sustainable source of energy. Including healthy fats, such as nuts, seeds, avocados, and olive oil, in your pre-workout meal can provide a sustained level of energy while sparing glycogen stores.

5.1.2 Micronutrients and Hydration: Supporting Factors in Pre-Workout Nutrition

While macronutrients provide the body with fuel, micronutrients play critical roles in supporting various physiological functions. Consuming essential vitamins and minerals during pre-workout helps in prepar

- **Vitamins and Minerals**
  B vitamins are especially vital for athletes, as they help in converting carbohydrates and fats into energy. Including food sources like whole grains, dark leafy greens, and dairy products can offer appropriate levels of B vitamins before a workout.
  Minerals like calcium, magnesium, and potassium are necessary for proper muscle function and regulating fluid balance. Dairy products, leafy greens, nuts, and seeds are good sources of these minerals and can be included in the pre-workout meal to support optimal performance.
- **Hydration**
  Adequate hydration before a workout is essential to maintain peak performance throughout the exercise session. Dehydration can result in fatigue, reduced stamina, and increased risk of injury. Drinking approximately 16 - 32 ounces of water, 2 - 3 hours before a workout, followed by an additional 8 ounces 20 - 30 minutes before the exercise begins can ensure optimal hydration levels.

5.1.3 Timing and Personalization: Fine-Tuning Your Pre-Workout Nutrition

The timing of your pre-workout meal holds significant importance in ensuring the body is sufficiently fueled for the exercise.

- **Timing**
  It is generally ideal to consume a balanced meal containing carbohydrates, proteins, and fats, approximately 3 - 4 hours before a workout. For athletes with busy schedules or those who prefer eating closer to the workout, a small snack containing simple carbohydrates and fast-digesting proteins can be consumed 30 - 60 minutes before exercise.
- **Personalization**
  Keep in mind that individual preferences and body requirements can differ. So, it's essential to understand and listen to your body and make adjustments according to your specific needs, exercise types, and overall goals.

In conclusion, pre-workout nutrition is a significant factor in optimizing performance, ensuring high energy levels, and promoting muscle recovery. Following a well-timed, balanced pre-workout meal can prove to be a game-changer when it comes to achieving optimal results from your workouts.

5.1 The Importance of Pre-Workout Nutrition

For an athlete, the importance of fueling the body before a workout or competition cannot be overstated. Pre-workout nutrition is essential for priming the body to perform at its best, enhance endurance, and reduce the risk of injury. In this section, we will discuss the functions of pre-workout nutrition and the ideal macronutrient composition which can be tailored to the needs of each athlete.

5.1.1 Functions of Pre-Workout Nutrition

Pre-workout nutrition serves several key purposes in preparing the body for optimal athletic performance:

1. **Energy Supply**: Proper nutrition ensures that the body has enough energy and nutrients to perform at its best. Consuming the right combination of carbohydrates, proteins, and fats provides the necessary fuel for the intended activity.
2. **Preserve Muscle Mass**: Pre-workout nutrition can help minimize muscle damage and breakdown during exercise. Consuming protein prior to a workout can supply the body with amino acids necessary to repair muscle tissue during and after exercise.
3. **Stabilize Blood Sugar Levels**: Eating pre-workout meals can help stabilize blood sugar levels, which is particularly important for endurance athletes who may be exercising for several hours. Low blood sugar levels can cause dizziness, fatigue, and poor performance.
4. **Proper Hydration**: Ensuring that the body is properly hydrated before engaging in any physical activity is crucial. Dehydration can lead to poor performance, muscle cramps, and increased risk of muscle injury.

5.1.2 Macronutrient Composition of Pre-Workout Meals

A well-balanced pre-workout meal should contain the following macronutrients:

1. **Carbohydrates**: Carbohydrates are the body's primary source of energy and should make up a

significant portion of an athlete's pre-workout meal. They provide the body with glucose, which is necessary for high-intensity exercise. Selecting complex carbohydrates such as whole grains, fruits, and vegetables will ensure a slow and steady release of energy throughout the workout.

2. **Protein**: Protein is essential for muscle growth and repair, making it a vital component of pre-workout nutrition. Consuming protein, particularly those rich in the amino acid leucine, can help stimulate muscle protein synthesis and reduce exercise-induced muscle damage. Good protein sources to consume prior to a workout include lean meats, dairy products, and plant-based protein sources like legumes and soy.

3. **Fats**: While fats have a relatively minor role in pre-workout nutrition, they shouldn't be ignored altogether. Consuming healthy fats like avocados, nuts, and olive oil can help provide additional energy for longer-duration, low-to-moderate intensity exercises. However, it is important to avoid consuming large amounts of fat before a workout, as it can slow down the digestion process and cause discomfort during exercise.

5.1.3 Timing and Portion Size

The timing of pre-workout nutrition is crucial for maximizing its benefits. Generally, a meal should be consumed 2-4 hours before exercising, providing ample time for digestion and absorption of nutrients. If a full meal isn't possible, a smaller snack can be eaten closer to the workout start, ideally within 30-60 minutes.

Portion size may vary based on an athlete's size, energy expenditure, and type of activity. Competitive endurance athletes, for example, may require larger pre-workout meals with higher carbohydrate content compared to those engaging in shorter-duration or lower-intensity exercise. Experimenting with different meal sizes and compositions can help determine what works best for each individual.

5.1.4 Sample Pre-Workout Meals

Here are some examples of balanced pre-workout meals to get you started:

1. Whole grain toast with almond butter and banana slices
2. Greek yogurt with granola and berries
3. A smoothie made with spinach, berries, protein powder, and almond milk
4. Brown rice or quinoa with lean chicken, steamed vegetables, and avocado
5. Oatmeal with chopped nuts, fruit, and a scoop of protein powder

In conclusion, the importance of pre-workout nutrition for optimal athletic performance cannot be overstated. Athletes should focus on consuming a balanced meal consisting of complex carbohydrates, protein, and healthy fats to fuel their bodies for the demands of their training or competition. Proper hydration is also crucial to prevent dehydration and decrease the risk of injury. Experiment with different meal compositions and timings to find the best strategy that works for you and supports your performance goals.

5.1 The Importance of Pre-Workout Nutrition

Performing at your best starts with fueling your body properly. The pre-workout meal is an essential part of any athletic routine because it provides the necessary energy, optimizes performance, and minimizes muscle damage. While the significance of post-workout nutrition is often emphasized, it is just as important to understand the role pre-workout nutrition plays in contributing to athletic success.

5.1.1 Balancing Macronutrients for Pre-Workout Fuel

A well-rounded pre-workout meal should include a balance of protein, carbohydrates, and fat to ensure optimal energy levels.

- **Protein:** Consuming adequate protein before a workout helps reduce muscle damage during exercise and aids in muscle recovery. Aim for 15-30 grams of protein one to three hours before your workout. Some sources include lean meats, fish, eggs, dairy products, or plant-based options like nuts, beans, and tofu.
- **Carbohydrates:** Carbohydrates are the primary fuel source during high-intensity exercise. Consuming 30-60 grams of carbohydrates before a workout helps improve endurance and overall performance. Opt for complex carbohydrates like whole grains, fruits, and vegetables, which provide longer-lasting energy.
- **Fat:** Although fat is not the primary energy source during high-intensity exercise, consuming moderate amounts in the pre-workout meal contributes to sustained energy levels during long workouts. Examples of healthy fats include avocados, nuts and seeds, olive oil, and fatty fish.

5.1.2 Timing Your Pre-Workout Nutrition

Consuming a carefully balanced meal two to four hours before your workout allows enough time for digestion and absorption of essential nutrients, ensuring optimal energy levels throughout the workout. Athletes with busy schedules who need a convenient and quick solution can also benefit from a pre-workout snack consisting of easily digestible foods 30 to 60 minutes before exercise. Some examples of such snacks include a piece of fruit, a granola bar, or a smoothie.

5.1.3 Hydration and Electrolytes

Proper hydration is critical for athletic performance. Begin hydrating several hours before your workout, aiming for at least 16-20 ounces of water during the 2-3 hours before exercise, and an additional 7-10 ounces in the 20-30 minutes leading up to your workout. Besides water, replenishing electrolytes, such as sodium, potassium, and magnesium, is important, especially during long or high-intensity workouts. You can find electrolyte-rich drinks or snacks to consume, or opt for natural sources such as fruits, vegetables, and nuts.

5.1.4 Supplements for Enhanced Performance

Certain supplements can help athletes improve their performance during workouts.

- **Caffeine:** Caffeine is a well-known stimulant that can increase energy levels, focus, endurance, and fat oxidation. Consume 3-6 milligrams of caffeine per kilogram of body weight about 30-60 minutes before a workout for optimal results.
- **Creatine:** Creatine is an amino acid that helps increase the body's ability to produce energy during high-intensity exercise. It can also aid in muscle

growth, strength, and recovery post-workout. Opt for 5-20 grams per day, with a loading phase of 20 grams daily for five days, followed by a maintenance phase of 5 grams per day.
- **Beta-Alanine:** This amino acid can help increase muscle carnosine levels, which aids in buffering acidity within the muscles during high-intensity exercise. Aim for 2-5 grams of beta-alanine daily for optimal results.

Remember to consult a healthcare professional when considering supplement usage. Not all supplements are applicable or suitable for every athlete or exercise goal.

5.1.5 Individualizing Your Pre-Workout Nutrition Plan

Keep in mind that every athlete is unique when it comes to nutritional needs and workout preferences. The timing and content of your pre-workout meal should be adjusted according to personal preferences, exercise intensity, and duration. Consider trial and error as you work through different macronutrient combinations, timings, and portion sizes to determine the optimal pre-workout meal plan that works best for you.

In conclusion, pre-workout nutrition plays a vital role in optimizing athletic performance. By creating a well-rounded meal plan that includes a balance of protein, carbohydrates, and fats, you can provide your body with the necessary fuel for high-intensity workouts. Additionally, maintain proper hydration and consider the use of supplements to enhance your overall performance further. Understanding the basics of pre-workout nutrition can mean the difference between merely going through the motions during your workout and pushing your limits to achieve peak performance.

5.1 Importance of Pre-Workout Nutrition

5.1.1 Overview

Pre-workout nutrition is a crucial component of an athlete's performance strategy. The goal of proper pre-workout nutrition is to provide the body with the proper nutrients, including carbohydrates, proteins, and fats, to fuel activity and optimize overall performance. Energy demand, intensity, and duration of the upcoming exercise are essential factors to consider when tailoring pre-workout nutrition strategies. Additionally, individual differences among athletes, such as body composition and metabolic rate, also impact pre-workout nutritional requirements.

5.1.2 Macro and Micronutrient Composition of Pre-Workout Nutrition

5.1.2.1 Carbohydrates

Carbohydrates serve as the primary source of fuel for most physical activities, especially high-intensity exercises. They are quickly broken down in the body into glucose, releasing energy required for muscle contractions. Adequate carbohydrate consumption before a workout ensures that glycogen stores in the muscles are full, reducing the risk of premature fatigue and promoting optimal performance.

Complex carbohydrates, such as whole grains, vegetables, and legumes, should be the focus of pre-workout nutrition. These carbohydrate sources are slower to digest, providing a continuous source of energy for muscles during workouts. Pre-workout meals should ideally be consumed approximately 2-4 hours before exercising, allowing for adequate digestion.

5.1.2.2 Proteins

Protein is a building block for muscles, tendons, ligaments, and other tissues. Pre-workout protein consumption helps fuel muscles that are activated during exercise and can also promote muscle repair and reduce muscle damage following activity. High-quality protein sources, such as lean meats, fish, dairy, and plant-based options, should be included in pre-workout meals. Athletes should aim for roughly 20-40 grams of protein in their pre-workout meal.

5.1.2.3 Fats

While not the primary source of energy during high-intensity activities, fats still play a key role in overall energy production. Fats can be beneficial in providing the body with a sustained energy source during endurance training. Healthy fats, such as avocado, nuts, and olive oil, should be included in pre-workout meals, but in moderate quantities. Excessive fat consumption prior to workouts may cause digestive issues and impede performance.

5.1.2.4 Micronutrients

In addition to macronutrients, certain micronutrients also require consideration in pre-workout nutrition planning. Essential vitamins and minerals like vitamin C, calcium, and iron can improve muscle function, boost the immune system, and promote optimal bone health. Including a variety of colorful fruits and vegetables in pre-workout meals can help athletes achieve ample micronutrient intake.

5.1.3 Hydration

Proper hydration is also critical for peak athletic performance. Dehydration can impair cognitive function, increase the risk of injury, and decrease overall performance. Athletes should aim to consume approximately 500-600 ml of water 2-3 hours prior to exercise and an additional 250-300 ml approximately 20-30 minutes before starting physical activity.

5.1.4 Special Considerations for Pre-Workout Nutrition

5.1.4.1 Timing of Pre-Workout Meals

As previously mentioned, pre-workout meals should ideally be consumed 2-4 hours prior to exercise. This timeframe allows for adequate digestion and absorption of nutrients, ensuring energy availability during workouts. If consuming a meal this far in advance is not possible, a smaller meal or easily digestible snack, such as a banana or a handful of almonds, should be consumed approximately 30-40 minutes before exercise.

5.1.4.2 Individual Variability

It is crucial to understand that each athlete is unique and therefore may respond differently to certain pre-workout nutrition strategies. Factors such as age, sex, body composition, and daily energy expenditure can influence nutritional needs. Therefore, working with a sports dietitian or nutritionist to create a personalized pre-workout nutrition plan is highly recommended.

5.1.4.3 Specific Sports or Exercise

Different sports and exercises require specific nutritional considerations based on factors such as intensity, duration, and required skill sets. For instance, endurance athletes like marathon runners or cyclists require more carbohydrates, while strength athletes, such as weight lifters, may benefit from higher protein intake. Addressing these specific needs is essential for optimizing pre-workout nutrition.

In conclusion, pre-workout nutrition plays an essential role in an athlete's overall performance strategy. Consuming adequate macronutrients, micronutrients, and hydration can result in increased energy availability, improved muscle function, and reduced fatigue during physical activity. Tailoring pre-workout nutrition to meet individual needs and specific sport demands can go a long way in enhancing athletic performance.

5.1 Timing and Composition: Keys to Optimal Pre-Workout Nutrition

5.1.1 Timing of Pre-Workout Meals

The timing of your pre-workout meal is crucial to ensure that your muscles have the necessary energy to perform at their best. As a general rule, consume a meal 3-4 hours before exercising to allow for digestion and absorption of nutrients. Below are more specific time frames to consider:

- **3-4 hours prior**: This is the window for your main pre-workout meal, which should be high in carbohydrates and moderate in protein. If you can't eat a large meal, consuming a smaller, carbohydrate-rich snack 30-60 minutes prior to your workout can also be effective in providing energy.
- **30-60 minutes prior**: While waiting until the last minute to eat may not be ideal, consuming a small,

easily digestible snack rich in carbohydrates and minimal in fiber, fat, and protein can provide a quick energy boost. Opt for a piece of fruit, a sports drink, or an energy gel.

5.1.2 Composition of Pre-Workout Meals

Carbohydrates

Carbohydrates are your body's primary fuel source during high-intensity exercise. Consuming carbohydrates before exercise can increase muscle glycogen stores, potentially delaying fatigue and improving performance. Research suggests aiming for approximately 1-4 grams of carbohydrates per kilogram of body weight within the 1-4 hours leading up to exercise.

Examples of carbohydrate-rich foods to incorporate into your pre-workout meal include:

- Rice, pasta, or potatoes
- Bread and bagels
- Fruit and fruit juices
- Oatmeal and cereals
- Quinoa

Protein

Protein consumption before exercise can help support muscle repair and growth. Aim to consume 0.25-0.4 grams of protein per kilogram of body weight within the 1-4 hours before your workout. While protein is an essential component of your pre-workwork nutrition, avoid prioritizing protein over carbohydrates, as this might hinder performance.

Examples of protein-rich foods to incorporate into your pre-workout meal include:

- Lean chicken or turkey
- Fish such as salmon or tuna
- Greek yogurt or cottage cheese
- Beans, lentils, or chickpeas
- Protein shakes (low-fat)

Fats

Fats are also an essential component of your pre-workout meal. However, limit your fat intake to a moderate level, as fatty foods tend to remain in the stomach for longer periods, which may cause gastrointestinal distress during exercise. Choose healthy sources of fat, such as whole food sources:

- Nuts and seeds (e.g., almonds, walnuts, chia seeds)
- Avocado
- Olive or canola oil
- Nut butters (e.g., almond or peanut butter)

Hydration

Proper hydration before exercise is key to prevent dehydration and optimize performance. Aim to drink 500-600 ml (approximately 17-20 ounces) of water 2-3 hours before exercise and an additional 300 ml (roughly 10 ounces) within 20-30 minutes of starting your workout.

5.1.3 Tailoring Pre-Workout Nutrition to Individual Needs and Preferences

Each athlete is unique, and pre-workout nutrition should be customized based on individual needs, preferences, and goals. Factors such as age, body composition, training intensity, and duration, as well as specific sport requirements, can affect your nutritional needs pre-exercise. Experimenting with different food combinations and timings is key to identifying the best pre-workout nutrition regimen that works for you.

5.1.4 Sample Pre-Workout Meals

Here are some sample pre-workout meal ideas for different scenarios:

3-4 Hours Prior (Main Pre-Workout Meal):

1. Brown rice, grilled chicken, and steamed vegetables with a small side of avocado.
2. Whole-grain pasta with marinara sauce, lean ground turkey, and a side of mixed green salad.
3. Quinoa with baked salmon, roasted chickpeas, and sautéed kale.

30-60 Minutes Prior (Quick Pre-Workout Snack):

1. Banana with 1-2 tablespoons of peanut butter.
2. Low-fat plain yogurt with a handful of berries.
3. Rice cake with a small spread of almond butter and sliced strawberries.

Remember, these are just a starting point. The most important aspect is to find what works best for you and your body's needs. Experiment with different foods and timings to develop your ideal pre-workout nutrition plan that sets you up for success.

6. Post-Workout Recovery: Replenishing and Repairing the Body

6.1 The Importance of Post-Workout Nutrition for Recovery

For athletes, understanding the connection between post-workout nutrition and recovery is of utmost importance. This critical period, immediately following a training session, is the time when the body seeks to repair the damage caused at the cellular level during exercise. This damage can occur in the form of muscle tears, glycogen depletion, and other metabolic stresses. It is also during this time that the body begins the process of adaptation, making it stronger and more capable to handle increased stress in the future.

To restore energy balance, replenish glycogen stores, and repair damaged muscle tissue, athletes must provide their bodies with the necessary nutrients. This can be done through a combination of macronutrients (protein, carbohydrates, and fats), along with micronutrients (vitamins and minerals).

6.1.1 Protein: The Building Block for Muscle Repair and Growth

After a workout, muscle proteins are physically damaged and need to be repaired. This damage signals the body to initiate muscle protein synthesis (MPS), a physiological process that involves the repair and rebuilding of muscle tissues. The rate at which this process occurs depends on several factors such as the type of exercise, individual levels of training, and nutrition.

During this recovery period, the body requires an adequate intake of dietary protein to provide the essential amino acids needed for MPS. Consuming protein post-workout has been shown to stimulate MPS, reduce muscle soreness, and enhance recovery. The International Society of Sports Nutrition recommends consuming 20-40 grams of high-quality protein within an hour following resistance training.

6.1.2 Carbohydrates: Replenishing Energy Stores to Fuel Performance

Intense or prolonged exercise depletes the body's glycogen stores which serve as its primary energy source. Replenishing these stores is important for instigating muscle repair and preventing excessive muscle breakdown. It has also been demonstrated that the consumption of carbohydrates post-workout can boost glycogen synthesis and accelerate recovery processes.

A common guideline is to consume 0.5-0.7 grams of carbohydrates per pound of body weight within 30 minutes post-exercise for optimal glycogen re-synthesis. The actual amount may vary depending on factors such as the intensity and duration of the exercise, as well as individual preferences.

6.1.3 Fats: Supporting Hormonal and Anti-Inflammatory Responses

While the focus of post-workout nutrition often lies on protein and carbohydrates, fats also play a beneficial role in recovery. They help modulate hormone production (e.g., testosterone) and provide essential fatty acids that combat inflammation, promote muscle growth, and support overall recovery. However, it is important not to over-consume fats immediately following a workout, as they can slow the absorption of carbohydrates and proteins. A moderate amount of healthy fats, such as those from nuts, seeds, or avocados, should be incorporated into a post-workout meal to support optimal recovery.

6.1.4 Micronutrients: Vitamins and Minerals for Optimal Recovery

In addition to macronutrients, certain vitamins and minerals play crucial roles in recovery processes. For example, electrolytes like sodium, potassium, and magnesium lost during sweating need to be replaced to aid fluid balance and prevent muscle cramps. Antioxidants, such as vitamins C and E, can help reduce exercise-induced oxidative stress and inflammation. Also, vitamin D and calcium are necessary for bone health and injury prevention.

To ensure an adequate intake of these nutrients post-workout, incorporating a variety of whole foods like fruits, vegetables, whole grains, and lean proteins is recommended. In some cases, supplementation may be necessary, but it is important to consult with a sports dietitian or other qualified professionals for individual guidance.

6.2 Timing and Strategies for Post-Workout Nutrition

To facilitate recovery and maintain performance, athletes should establish specific post-workout nutrition strategies that cater to their unique needs, preferences, and circumstances. The effectiveness of these strategies largely depends on nutrient timing and the type of workout performed.

6.2.1 The Anabolic Window: Maximizing Recovery and Adaptation

The so-called "anabolic window" refers to the period immediately following exercise when the body is primed to absorb nutrients in order to fuel recovery and adaptation. Consuming a combination of protein and carbohydrates during this window facilitates muscle protein synthesis, reduces muscle soreness, and replenishes glycogen stores. While research suggests that nutrients are more effectively absorbed within the first hour post-workout, recent studies have shown that these benefits can still be attained within a broader time frame, up to several hours after exercise. However, it is generally recommended to consume a meal containing a balance of macronutrients within one to two hours of training.

6.2.2 Post-Workout Nutrition Based on Exercise Type

The composition of a post-workout meal should be tailored to the specific demands of the exercise performed. For instance, following high-intensity or prolonged endurance workouts, higher amounts of carbohydrates may be required to replenish glycogen stores. On the other hand, following resistance training or activities that place a greater emphasis on muscle building, higher protein intake may be more favorable. Finally, it is important to consider the role of rest days or lower-intensity workouts, where the focus should be on supporting overall recovery, ensuring adequate hydration, and maintaining balanced nutrient intake.

6.3 Example Post-Workout Meals

Finding effective post-workout meal options can be a matter of individual preference, dietary restrictions, and accessibility. Here are some examples of balanced post-workout meals:

1. Grilled chicken with roasted vegetables (e.g., sweet potatoes or broccoli)
2. Whole grain toast topped with mashed avocado, turkey breast, and tomato slices
3. Greek yogurt with mixed berries, honey, and a handful of almonds
4. Smoothie made with protein powder, mixed fruits, spinach, and almond milk
5. Rice bowl with beans, mixed greens, avocado, and salsa

In conclusion, understanding the science behind post-workout nutrition can significantly improve an athlete's ability to recover and perform at their best. By ensuring an adequate intake of proteins, carbohydrates, fats, and micronutrients, athletes can facilitate muscle repair, replenish glycogen stores, and support the body in its adaptation to increased physical demands. Developing individualized post-workout nutrition strategies based on exercise type and personal preferences can help lay the foundation for long-term success in athletic pursuits.

6.1 The Importance of Post-Workout Nutrition

After an intense workout, the body enters a phase of recovery and repair, where post-workout nutrition plays a critical role in determining the success and quality of that recovery. Properly refueling your body with the right nutrients helps to:

1. Maximize muscle repair and growth
2. Replenish energy stores, such as glycogen
3. Improve overall workout performance in the long term
4. Promote optimal adaptation to exercise and reduce injury risks

During exercises, our muscles go through a series of microscopic damages and experience a significant depletion of energy stores, especially glycogen. To replenish the energy and repair those damages, it is important to consume the right nutrients soon enough after the workout. These nutrients include carbohydrates, protein, and hydration in the form of water or electrolyte-based drinks.

6.1.1 Carbohydrates: Restoring Energy and Supporting Muscle Growth

Carbohydrates are the primary fuel source for energy when it comes to exercise. During a workout, the body taps into glycogen stores found in the liver and muscles. Glycogen fuels the body's energy needs during high-intensity exercises. Depleted glycogen stores can lead to decreased energy levels and negatively impact your workout performance. After a workout, consuming carbohydrates helps replenish glycogen stores and support muscle repair by increasing insulin levels, which can promote muscle growth.

The ideal time to consume carbohydrates is within 30 minutes to 2 hours after the workout, with a recommended intake of 0.5-0.7 grams of carbohydrates per pound of body weight. Consuming carbohydrates alongside protein can help maximize glycogen stores and promote muscle growth. For athletes who train multiple times a day, refueling glycogen stores quickly is especially important to maintain and improve performance levels.

Examples of high-quality carbohydrate sources include:

- Whole grains like brown rice, quinoa, and whole wheat bread
- Fruits such as bananas, apples, and berries
- Starchy vegetables like potatoes, sweet potatoes, and corn
- Legumes and beans

6.1.2 Protein: Repairing and Rebuilding Muscles

During a workout, especially resistance training, some proteins in the muscles get damaged, producing microscopic tears in muscle fibers. Consuming protein post-workout helps trigger muscle protein synthesis, which repairs the damaged tissues, promotes the creation of new muscle tissues, and fosters hypertrophy (i.e., muscle growth). Protein intake also positively influences glycogen restoration and reduces muscle soreness after exercise.

Depending on the intensity and duration of the exercise, protein requirements can vary from approximately 15–30 grams of protein post-workout for ideal muscle recovery. It is crucial to consume a complete protein source, containing all the essential amino acids. The combination of essential amino acids, especially leucine, is necessary to maximize muscle protein synthesis.

Examples of high-quality protein sources include:

- Lean meats such as chicken, turkey, and lean cuts of beef
- Fish and seafood like salmon, tuna, and shrimp
- Dairy products such as Greek yogurt, cottage cheese, and milk
- Plant-based options like tofu, tempeh, and edamame
- Protein shakes and bars with minimal added sugars

6.1.3 Hydration: Restoring Fluid Balance and Supporting Recovery

Maintaining proper hydration is crucial for optimal post-workout recovery. During exercise, your body loses water and electrolytes, such as sodium and potassium, through sweat. Intense workouts can lead to significant fluid loss, which can negatively impact recovery time, athletic performance, and even increase the risk of injury.

For maximal recovery, the athletes should aim to replace the fluids lost during exercise. As a general rule, you should consume 16-24 ounces of water for every pound lost during exercise. Sports drinks containing electrolytes can also be useful if your workout session was long and intense, lasting more than an hour.

In addition to water, some fruits and vegetables – like watermelon, cucumber, and oranges – can provide you with extra hydration and electrolytes.

6.1.4 Putting It All Together: The Ideal Post-Workout Meal

Timing, quality, and balance of nutrients are all important factors to consider for an ideal post-workout meal. A combination of carbohydrates and protein consumed within

30 minutes to 2 hours after a workout can significantly improve recovery and overall performance.

To create an effective post-workout meal, include:

1. High-quality carbohydrates, such as fruits, whole grains, or starchy vegetables
2. Protein from lean meats, fish, dairy, or plant-based sources
3. Plenty of water or an electrolyte-rich sports drink, if needed

Some examples of post-workout meals include:

- Grilled chicken breast with brown rice and steamed vegetables
- Protein shake with banana, spinach, and almond milk
- Greek yogurt with berries and a drizzle of honey

In conclusion, investing the time and effort into properly nourishing your body post-workout is essential for achieving long-lasting results, maximizing recovery, and supporting your overall athletic performance. Prioritizing carbohydrates, protein, and hydration in your post-workout nutrition will improve muscle growth, restore energy stores, optimize performance, and reduce injury risks.

6.1 The Importance of Post-Workout Recovery Nutrition

6.1.1 Introduction

Post-workout recovery is a critical component of any athlete's training regimen. Adequate recovery is essential for repairing damaged muscles, maintaining peak physical performance, and preventing injuries. Proper nutrition is crucial for ensuring the body is adequately replenished and repaired after exercise. This subsection highlights the importance of post-workout recovery nutrition, outlining the key nutrients and strategies that athletes need to include in their diet to speed up recovery and optimize results.

6.1.2 The Three R's of Recovery Nutrition: Rehydrate, Refuel, and Repair

To maximize post-workout recovery, athletes should focus on the three R's - rehydrate, refuel, and repair. These components aim to restore fluids and electrolytes lost through sweat, replenish glycogen stores, and repair muscle tissues to support strength and growth.

Rehydrate: Maintaining proper hydration during and after workouts is crucial for supporting essential bodily functions and preventing dehydration-related side effects such as fatigue, dizziness, and reduced cognitive function. Consuming at least 16-24 ounces of water for every pound lost during exercise, and sipping a sports drink containing electrolytes, can help athletes rehydrate efficiently.

Refuel: Intense exercise depletes glycogen stores in muscles, which is the body's primary source of energy during workouts. To replenish these energy stores, athletes should consume high-quality carbohydrates such as whole grains, fruits, and starchy vegetables within 30 minutes to 2 hours post-workout. The recommended intake is approximately 1.2 grams of carbohydrates per kilogram of body weight in the first hour, followed by an additional 1.2 grams per kilogram in the second hour.

Repair: During exercise, muscle tissues sustain damage, leading to a natural inflammatory response and triggering the need for repair and growth. To support muscle recovery, athletes should consume high-quality protein sources such as lean meats, dairy products, or plant-based proteins like legumes and tofu. Aim to consume 20-30 grams of protein within 30 minutes to 2 hours post-workout to promote optimal muscle protein synthesis, which is the process by which the body repairs and rebuilds muscle tissue.

6.1.3 Nutrient Timing: What and When to Eat for Optimal Recovery

While it is essential to consume adequate nutrients after exercise, the timing of nutrient intake also plays a vital role in maximizing recovery. Research suggests that there is a "window of opportunity" within the first 45 minutes to 2 hours post-workout when the body is primed to absorb nutrients for recovery and repair.

Carbohydrates: Consuming carbohydrates during the post-exercise window helps replenish glycogen stores quickly and effectively, which contributes to improved performance in subsequent training sessions. Studies indicate that athletes experience greater glycogen replenishment when they consume carbohydrates immediately after exercise rather than delaying intake.

Protein: Consuming protein within the post-exercise window is crucial for stimulating muscle protein synthesis, which is essential for muscle repair, growth, and adaptation. Incorporating both fast-absorbing proteins (e.g., whey protein) and slow-absorbing proteins (e.g., casein) can optimize muscle repair throughout the recovery period.

Combination of Carbohydrates and Protein: Studies have shown that the simultaneous consumption of carbohydrates and protein during the post-workout recovery window can enhance glycogen synthesis, muscle protein synthesis, and reduce muscle soreness. Aim for a ratio of 31 or 41 carbohydrates to protein for optimal recovery, such as chocolate milk, Greek yogurt with honey and berries, or whole-grain bread with lean meat.

6.1.4 Micronutrients and Antioxidants for Recovery

While carbohydrates, proteins, and fluids are the primary focus of post-workout recovery nutrition, several micronutrients and antioxidants also play a critical role in supporting overall health, reducing inflammation, and aiding in recovery.

Vitamins and Minerals: Vitamins such as B-complex vitamins, vitamin D, and minerals such as calcium, magnesium, and iron are essential for post-workout recovery. These micronutrients support energy production, electrolyte balance, bone health, and various other cellular processes. Consuming a balanced diet including dairy products, leafy green vegetables, and lean meats will help meet the daily recommended amounts.

Antioxidants: Exercise-induced muscle damage and inflammation can be mitigated by including antioxidant-rich foods in the post-workout meal. Antioxidants such as vitamin C, vitamin E, and polyphenols found in fruits, vegetables, and green tea can help combat oxidative stress caused by exercise, supporting muscle recovery and overall health.

6.1.5 Conclusion

Post-workout recovery nutrition plays a pivotal role in supporting optimal athletic performance, preventing injuries, and improving overall health. Incorporating the three R's of recovery – rehydrate, refuel, and repair – along with the proper timing of nutrient intake and inclusion of micronutrients and antioxidants in the diet will help athletes make the most of their training efforts and reach their full potential.

Understanding and implementing these strategies will enable athletes to experience accelerated muscle recovery, reduced soreness, and improved performance, leading to enhanced athletic success and longevity in their chosen sports.

6. Post-Workout Recovery: Replenishing and Repairing the Body

6.1. The Golden Hour: Why Post-Workout Nutrition Matters

After completing an intensive workout, there is a critical 45-60 minute window – commonly referred to as the "golden hour" (Jentjens & Jeukendrup, 2003) – during which the body's ability to absorb and utilize nutrients to maximize recovery is at its peak. This is due to increased blood flow and enzyme activity within the muscles, which accelerates nutrient absorption, glycogen synthesis, and protein synthesis (Ivy et al., 2002).

Since workouts break down muscle fibers, and your glycogen stores (the body's primary source of energy) are depleted, it is crucial to address both of these issues immediately after exercising. The three major nutrition components that play a crucial role in post-workout recovery are protein, carbohydrates, and hydration.

6.2. Protein Power: Repairing Damaged Muscle Fibers

During a workout, muscle fibers undergo microtrauma – tiny tears that need to be repaired for muscle growth to occur. Consuming protein in the post-workout period provides the necessary amino acids to repair these damaged fibers, promote muscle protein synthesis, and prevent muscle breakdown (Macnaughton et al., 2016).

The ideal amount of protein to consume post-workout varies depending on factors such as body weight, training intensity, and individual needs, with a general guideline being 20-30 grams of high-quality protein within 30 minutes of your workout (Kerksick et al., 2017).

Some quick and convenient sources of high-quality protein post-workout include:

- Whey protein powder
- Greek yogurt or cottage cheese
- Lean meats such as chicken, turkey, or fish
- Plant-based proteins such as tofu, tempeh, or a plant-based protein powder

6.3. Carbohydrate Replenishment: Restoring Energy Stores

In addition to protein, consuming sufficient carbohydrates is necessary to replenish glycogen stores and support muscle recovery. Carbohydrates provide glucose, which the body uses to synthesize glycogen and replace the energy reserves lost during exercise (Burke et al., 2004).

The ideal amount of carbohydrates post-workout depends on the intensity and duration of your exercise, as well as your daily carbohydrate needs based on factors such as body weight and activity level. A general guideline is to consume

1.0-1.2g of carbohydrates per kilogram of body weight within 30 minutes of exercise (Kerksick et al., 2017).

Some examples of carbohydrate-rich post-workout foods include:

- Fresh or dried fruit
- Whole-grain bread, crackers, or pasta
- Starchy vegetables such as sweet potatoes, corn, or peas
- Low-fat dairy products such as milk or yogurt

6.4. Hydrate to Recover: The Importance of Fluid and Electrolyte Replacement

Hydration plays a crucial role in post-workout recovery, as the body loses fluid and electrolytes through sweat during exercise. Dehydration can impair muscle function, hinder recovery, and increase the risk of cramping and injury (Popkin et al., 2010).

To optimize hydration status post-workout, it is recommended to drink 500-1000ml of fluid within the first 30 minutes following exercise and continue consumption at regular intervals (Sawka et al., 2007). This should include water or sports drinks containing electrolytes such as sodium, potassium, and magnesium, which are essential for proper muscle function and fluid balance.

6.5. Putting it All Together: Post-Workout Meal Ideas

To maximize the benefits of post-workout nutrition, try to consume a meal or snack containing both protein and carbohydrates within that crucial "golden hour". Below are some balanced post-workout meal ideas:

- Whole-grain turkey and cheese sandwich with a piece of fruit
- Protein smoothie with banana, spinach, and almond milk
- Greek yogurt with granola and mixed berries
- Chicken or tofu stir-fry with brown rice and vegetables

By prioritizing post-workout nutrition, athletes can optimize their recovery, improve their physical performance, and reduce the risk of injury. With a comprehensive understanding of the essential components of a post-workout meal and the timing of nutrient consumption, you can help your body repair and refuel effectively, ensuring that you are prepared and energized for your next performance.

6.1 Why Post-Workout Recovery is Integral to Athletic Success: The Science and What's at Stake

After an intense workout or an adrenaline-pumping athletic event, replenishment and repair of the body are essential for optimal recovery and maintaining the overall health and wellness of the athlete. There are three primary objectives that a post-workout recovery plan strives to fulfill:

1. Rehydrate: Replenishing lost fluids, electrolytes, and water is vital in preventing dehydration and maintaining physical health.
2. Refuel: Restoring depleted glycogen stores in the muscles to ensure their proper functioning during future training sessions and athletic events.
3. Repair: Providing essential nutrients to support the growth and repair of muscle tissues, ultimately

leading to increased muscle strength, mass, and athletic ability.

6.1.1 Understanding Glycogen

Glycogen is the stored form of glucose, serving as a primary source of energy that fuels the body during physical activities. The glycogen reserves are mainly situated in the muscles and liver. When the body's energy levels are running low, glycogen is broken down into glucose to be utilized by working muscles, keeping the body supported during short bursts of intense activity, such as sprinting or weight lifting.

However, these glycogen stores get depleted during these high-intensity physical activities. Inadequate replenishment of these reserves can lead to a decline in athletic performance and an increased likelihood of injury.

6.1.2 The Significance of Hydration

Fluid loss from sweating during exercise can cause dehydration due to an imbalance in the body's water content. Maintaining proper hydration levels is crucial for various physiological processes, such as thermoregulation, blood transport of nutrients, and maintaining an electrolyte balance that aids in muscle contraction and performance. After a workout, replacing these lost fluids is necessary to restore the body to its optimal state.

6.1.3 The Role of Protein in Muscle Recovery and Repair

Protein is a vital component of not only post-workout recovery but also overall well-being for athletes. It's a macronutrient consisting of chains of amino acids that provide essential functions, including repairing and building new muscle tissue. Intense workouts and prolonged physical activities stress and damage muscle fibers. In response, the body signals muscle protein synthesis to repair these micro-tears, resulting in an increase in muscle mass and overall strength.

Consuming adequate amounts of protein after a workout ensures that the body has the essential amino acids required to carry out the growth and repair processes.

6.1.4 The Importance of Macronutrient Timing

The timing of nutrient consumption, as well as the types of nutrients ingested, are key factors to consider for athletes attempting to maximize their post-workout recovery. Research has shown that there is a "window of opportunity" (approximately 30-45 minutes) after a workout when the body is most receptive to repair and refueling. During this time frame, the consumption of carbohydrates and protein in the right proportions can facilitate the most effective post-workout recovery.

6.1.5 Macronutrient Ratios for Optimal Post-Workout Recovery

While individual needs may vary, the general consensus among nutrition experts is that a combination of carbohydrates and protein can provide the ideal composition for post-workout recovery. A widely recommended ratio is 3:1 of carbohydrates to protein, with a focus on higher quality sources, such as complex carbohydrates and complete proteins.

For example, an athlete may consume a meal or snack containing:

- 60 g of carbohydrates (3 portions) from whole grains, fruits, or vegetables
- 20 g of protein (1 portion) from lean meat, fish, eggs, dairy or plant-based sources like beans and legumes

An ultimate post-workout recovery strategy would combine adequate hydration with a balanced intake of carbohydrates and protein to maximize the replenishment of energy stores, support muscle recovery, and enhance athletic performance.

6.2 Post-Workout Recovery Supplements and their Efficacy

Post-workout supplements may offer an efficient and convenient way to meet the required macronutrient needs of athletes for optimal recovery. However, it's crucial to evaluate the scientific evidence behind these supplements to ensure that they are effective and safe.

6.2.1 Protein Powders

Protein powders, such as whey, casein, and plant-based sources (e.g., soy, pea or rice protein), have gained prominence due to their portable and easy-to-consume format. Some studies have found that consuming protein powders post-workout may enhance muscle protein synthesis and aid recovery. However, athletes should prioritize whole food sources of protein over supplements and consume protein powders only if they cannot meet their recovery needs through whole foods alone.

6.2.2 Branch Chain Amino Acids (BCAAs)

BCAAs are a group of three amino acids—leucine, isoleucine, and valine—that play a crucial role in muscle protein synthesis. Supplementation with BCAAs has been suggested to reduce muscle damage, alleviate muscle soreness, and improve endurance. However, recent studies have concluded that consuming complete proteins containing all nine essential amino acids (EAAs) may be more beneficial for muscle recovery and growth than just BCAAs.

6.2.3 Creatine

Creatine is an organic compound found in muscle cells that plays a role in producing energy during high-intensity activities. Supplementation with creatine has been shown to increase strength and power output during short-duration, high-intensity exercise, potentially enhancing performance in sports like weightlifting and sprinting. While creatine has limited direct effects on post-workout recovery, it can contribute to overall athletic performance.

While post-workout supplements may aid in recovery for some athletes, the primary focus should be on consuming a balanced diet that provides all necessary macronutrients and micronutrients. Supplements should be considered only as an adjunct to a well-rounded, whole-food-based diet.

6.3 Building your Post-Workout Recovery Strategy: Practical Tips and Considerations

Incorporating specific post-workout nutrition strategies is an essential aspect of an athlete's overall nutrition plan. Here are some practical tips to optimize post-workout recovery:

- Plan your post-workout meal or snack in advance, ensuring it contains the appropriate macronutrient ratios, and is easily digestible to maximize nutrient absorption.
- Prioritize whole foods over supplements when possible, focusing on high-quality sources of carbohydrates and protein.
- Practice individualized portion control to cater to your unique recovery needs based on factors such as age, gender, bodyweight, the intensity of the workout, and training goals.
- Ensure adequate hydration before, during, and after your workout. Monitor your fluid intake and aim to replace fluid losses through sweat 1:1 with fluid consumption. In cases of significant electrolyte losses, opt for electrolyte-containing beverages such as sports drinks, coconut water, or even a homemade solution containing water, salt, and some fruit juice.
- Monitor your recovery progress frequently by tracking factors such as muscle soreness, energy levels, and athletic performance, and make adjustments to your recovery and nutrition plan as needed.

By understanding the science behind post-workout recovery and incorporating evidence-based strategies, athletes can maximize their healing, fuel their bodies more effectively, and ultimately see better results in training and competition.

7. Ergogenic Aids: Supplements and Performance Enhancers for Athletes

7.1 An Introduction to Ergogenic Aids: The Edge in Athletic Performance

Ergogenic aids refer to any external influences that can enhance an athlete's performance by improving their energy production or efficiency, increasing recovery rate, or reducing fatigue. They can come in various forms, including supplements, technology, and performance-enhancing substances. As an athlete striving to reach peak performance, understanding the science behind ergogenic aids can help you make informed decisions about what to include in your nutrition and training regimen.

The use of ergogenic aids has been a controversial topic in the sports world, with many debates regarding their safety, ethics, and effectiveness. Nonetheless, research on ergogenic aids continues to advance, providing valuable information for athletes and coaches alike. This chapter will guide you through the different types of ergogenic aids, their effects on athletic performance, and considerations to keep in mind when incorporating them into your routine.

7.1.1 Types of Ergogenic Aids

7.1.1.1 Nutritional Supplements

Nutritional supplements are products intended to supplement an athlete's diet and provide essential nutrients, such as vitamins, minerals, amino acids, and other functional food components. They may be particularly beneficial for athletes with dietary restrictions or those training at a high volume or intensity. Some common examples include:

- **Protein Powder:** A concentrated source of protein that can help support muscle growth and repair, particularly after intense training sessions.
- **Creatine Monohydrate:** A naturally occurring compound found in muscle tissue that can boost short-term anaerobic performance and support muscle strength and mass gains.
- **Beta-Alanine:** An amino acid that may improve exercise performance by enhancing the buffering capacity of muscles and delaying the onset of fatigue.
- **Branched-Chain Amino Acids (BCAAs):** A group of essential amino acids (leucine, isoleucine, and valine) that can support muscle recovery and reduce muscle breakdown during exercise.

7.1.1.2 Performance-Enhancing Substances

Performance-enhancing substances are chemicals or compounds that can improve athletic performance through a variety of mechanisms. They may be legally approved for use, such as caffeine or beetroot juice, or banned by regulatory bodies, such as anabolic steroids and blood doping. Some examples of performance-enhancing substances include:

- **Caffeine:** A stimulant that can enhance alertness, reduce fatigue, and improve endurance and power output.

- **Nitrates (found in Beetroot Juice):** Naturally occurring compounds that can improve endurance performance by enhancing blood flow and oxygen delivery to working muscles.
- **Beta-2 Agonists:** A class of drugs that can improve endurance and power output by relaxing airway muscles and increasing oxygen delivery to working muscles.
- **Erythropoietin (EPO):** A hormone that stimulates red blood cell production, enhancing oxygen delivery to working muscles, and improving endurance performance. EPO is generally considered a banned substance in most sports.

7.1.1.3 Technology and Equipment

Advancements in technology and equipment have given athletes access to novel ergogenic aids that can optimize their training and recovery. Examples include:

- **Compression Garments:** Clothing designed to provide graduated compression to enhance blood flow, reduce muscle soreness, and improve recovery.
- **Altitude Training and Hypoxic Tents:** Devices and environments that simulate high-altitude conditions to improve an athlete's oxygen-carrying capacity, ultimately enhancing endurance performance.
- **Whole Body Cryotherapy:** An emerging recovery method that involves short exposures to extremely cold temperatures, aimed at reducing inflammation and muscle soreness.

7.1.2 Factors to Consider When Using Ergogenic Aids

Before incorporating ergogenic aids into your training and nutrition plan, evaluate the following factors to ensure their optimal use:

- **Effectiveness:** Assess the quality and consistency of the scientific evidence supporting the ergogenic aid's claims. Look for peer-reviewed research from reputable sources, and understand that not all ergogenic aids will have the same impact on every athlete.
- **Safety:** Always prioritize your health and well-being. Some ergogenic aids may carry risks or side effects, so consult with a sports medicine professional or sports dietitian before using any new supplements or substances.
- **Legality:** Familiarize yourself with the regulations of your sport's governing body and anti-doping policies. Using banned substances may result in severe consequences, from disqualification to suspension or even legal repercussions.
- **Cost-Benefit Analysis:** Weigh the potential benefits of an ergogenic aid against its financial cost and the time and effort required to incorporate it into your routine.

In conclusion, ergogenic aids can offer a competitive edge for athletes, but using them safely and effectively requires a thorough understanding of the science behind each aid. As the field of sports nutrition continues to evolve and new ergogenic aids emerge, it's essential to stay informed and make informed decisions that align with your training goals and values.

7.1 Overview of Ergogenic Aids: Separating Science from Hype

Performance enhancement has always been the holy grail for athletes seeking a competitive edge. As sport becomes more competitive, seeking new and improved ways to optimize performance has become the key to success for many. One such area of interest is ergogenic aids, a term that encompasses a wide range of supplements and performance-enhancing products specifically designed to help athletes achieve their full potential. In this section, we will explore the various types of ergogenic aids, their proposed benefits, and the scientific evidence that supports (or refutes) their use.

7.1.1 What are Ergogenic Aids?

Ergogenic aids are any external factors that can improve athletic performance. These can include mechanical aids, such as specialized training equipment or the latest footwear technology, as well as more elusive aids like mental techniques for staying focused under pressure. The focus of this section, however, is on dietary supplements and other nutrient-based interventions, such as vitamins, minerals, herbs, and various other compounds, which are often marketed to athletes and casual exercisers as essential tools for optimizing performance and recovery.

7.1.2 Types of Ergogenic Aids: A Broad Overview

Ergogenic aids can be broadly categorized into four main groups:

1. **Nutritional Ergogenic Aids**: These are dietary supplements containing nutrients, vitamins, minerals, or other compounds that are purported to improve performance, aid in recovery, or support overall health. Examples include protein powders, amino acid supplements, creatine, and energy gels.

2. **Pharmacological Ergogenic Aids**: These include drugs and other pharmaceutical compounds that can have powerful effects on the body, such as improving muscle strength, reducing inflammation or promoting cardiovascular health. Examples include anabolic steroids, human growth hormone (HGH), erythropoietin (EPO), and beta-blockers. It is essential to note that many pharmacological ergogenic aids are banned in competitive sports due to their potential health risks and the unfair advantage they may provide.
3. **Physiological Ergogenic Aids**: These interventions manipulate the body's natural processes to improve athletic performance, typically by optimizing the body's use of oxygen or energy. Examples include blood doping, hyperbaric oxygen therapy, or altitude training.
4. **Psychological Ergogenic Aids**: These methods are designed to improve an athlete's mental state, focus, and concentration during competition. Examples include meditation, visualization, and the use of music or other audio stimuli to enhance mental performance or reduce stress.

7.1.3 Evaluating the Evidence: A Word of Caution

Given the immense marketing hype surrounding many ergogenic aids, it is essential to examine the scientific evidence behind their promises critically. Some products have a strong body of research supporting their efficacy, while others may be based on little more than anecdotal evidence or weak research.

Athletes should be aware of the potential risks and rewards when considering any ergogenic aid, supplement, or performance-enhancing substance. Consulting with a healthcare professional, such as a registered dietitian, sports nutritionist or sports medicine physician, can be extremely helpful in navigating the vast array of products and determining what may be suitable for an individual's unique needs and circumstances.

In the following sections, we will detail some of the most popular and widely researched ergogenic aids, exploring their proposed benefits, mechanisms of action, and the scientific evidence supporting their use.

7.2 Nutritional Ergogenic Aids: Popular Supplements and Their Evidence Base

7.2.1 Creatine

Proposed Benefits: Creatine is one of the most popular and well-researched ergogenic aids available. Studies have consistently shown that creatine supplementation, typically in the form of creatine monohydrate, can lead to improvements in strength, power, and muscle mass, particularly during high-intensity, short-duration activities such as weightlifting or sprinting.

Mechanism of Action: Creatine is naturally present in the body and plays a crucial role in energy production within muscle cells. Supplementation increases the levels of creatine within muscle tissue, which in turn allows for more rapid and efficient regeneration of adenosine triphosphate (ATP) – the primary source of energy for cellular processes – during bouts of high-intensity activity. This enhanced energy production can result in increased strength, power output, and muscle mass.

Evidence: There is a strong body of evidence indicating that creatine supplementation can result in significant improvements in various markers of athletic performance. A meta-analysis of over 30 studies concluded that creatine supplementation increases muscle strength by an average of 8%, muscle power by 14%, and sprint performance by 1-5% (1). While the effects of creatine are most pronounced in high-intensity, short-duration activities, some research also suggests that endurance athletes may experience modest benefits from supplementation, particularly when engaging in high-intensity intervals within their training programs (2).

7.2.2 Beta-Alanine

Proposed Benefits: Beta-alanine supplementation has been shown to improve high-intensity exercise performance, particularly during activities lasting 1-4 minutes, such as middle-distance running, swimming, or team sports.

Mechanism of Action: When ingested, beta-alanine combines with histidine to form carnosine – a naturally occurring dipeptide found primarily in skeletal muscle. Carnosine plays a critical role in regulating the acidity within muscle tissue during high-intensity exercise, which is a limiting factor in the onset of fatigue. By supplementing with beta-alanine, athletes can increase their muscle carnosine levels, delay the onset of fatigue, and perform at a higher intensity for more extended periods.

Evidence: A meta-analysis of 40 studies found that beta-alanine supplementation resulted in a small but significant improvement in exercise performance of 2.85% for tasks lasting between 1-4 minutes (3). Other research has noted that beta-alanine supplementation may be particularly beneficial for athletes involved in high-intensity interval training or repeated sprint activities (4).

7.2.3 Branched-Chain Amino Acids (BCAAs)

Proposed Benefits: BCAAs are widely used by athletes who believe that supplementation can improve exercise performance, support muscle growth and recovery, and minimize muscle soreness following high-intensity activity. The three primary BCAAs are leucine, isoleucine, and valine.

Mechanism of Action: BCAAs are essential amino acids, meaning they cannot be synthesized by the body and must be obtained from dietary sources. Several proposed mechanisms may explain the potential ergogenic benefits of BCAA supplementation, including reduced muscle protein breakdown during exercise, increased protein synthesis following exercise, and reduced perceived exertion during activity due to alterations in neurotransmitter levels in the brain.

Evidence: The research on BCAAs and exercise performance is somewhat mixed, with some studies suggesting little to no benefit for supplementation above the BCAAs provided through a balanced diet containing sufficient protein. A recent review of BCAA supplementation and exercise concluded that "the current evidence is insufficient to support the use of BCAA supplementation alone for the purpose of enhancing endurance or high-intensity exercise performance" (5). However, some evidence suggests that BCAA supplementation may play a role in reducing muscle soreness and improving recovery following high-intensity activity (6).

As with any supplement or ergogenic aid, it is crucial to critically evaluate the scientific evidence while considering individual factors such as goals, current dietary intake, and potential interactions with other supplements, medications, or health conditions. Always consult with a healthcare professional before making any substantial changes to your diet, supplement regimen or training intensity.

References

1. Branch JD. Effect of creatine supplementation on body composition and performance: a meta-analysis. Int J Sport Nutr Exerc Metab. 2003 Jun;13(2):198-226.
2. van Loon LJ, Oosterlaar AM, Hartgens F, Hesselink MK, Snow RJ, Wagenmakers AJ. Effects of creatine loading and prolonged creatine supplementation on body composition, fuel selection, sprint and endurance performance in humans. Clin Sci (Lond). 2003 Feb;104(2):153-62.
3. Hobson RM, Saunders B, Ball G, Harris RC, Sale C. Effects of β-alanine supplementation on exercise performance: a meta-analysis. Amino Acids. 2012 Jul;43(1):25-37.
4. Derave W, Özdemir MS, Harris RC, Pottier A, Reyngoudt H, Koppo K, Wise JA, Achten E. Beta-Alanine supplementation augments muscle carnosine content and attenuates fatigue during repeated isokinetic contraction bouts in trained sprinters. J Appl Physiol. 2007 Nov;103(5):1736-43.
5. Stevens BR, Godfrey MD, Kaminski TW, Braith RW. High-intensity dynamic human muscle performance enhanced by a metabolic intervention. Med Sci Sports Exerc. 2000 Dec;32(12):2102-8.
6. Jackman SR, Witard OC, Jeukendrup AE, Tipton KD. Branched-chain amino acid ingestion can ameliorate soreness from eccentric exercise. Med Sci Sports Exerc. 2010 May;42(5):962-70.

7.1 The Importance of Ergogenic Aids for Athletes

Ergogenic aids are any external factors or substances that can enhance an athlete's performance. The term "ergogenic" is derived from the Greek word "ergon", which means "work" and "genes," which means "born of." Therefore, ergogenic aids help athletes perform more work or physical activity. These aids can come in various forms: dietary supplements, performance-enhancing drugs, sports equipment, and other external factors that can influence an athlete's performance.

As an athlete, maintaining optimal health and achieving peak performance on the field often relies on the fine balance of their training regimen, nutrition, and proper recovery. Introducing ergogenic aids into one's routine can provide that extra edge needed to separate oneself from the competition. Thus, knowing and understanding various ergogenic aids can provide a significant advantage for athletes.

7.1.1 Types of Ergogenic Aids

The most common ergogenic aids can be classified into the following categories:

- **Nutritional Ergogenic Aids**: These are nutritional supplements that may help enhance an athlete's performance. Examples include creatine, caffeine, beta-alanine, and sodium bicarbonate.
- **Pharmacologic Ergogenic Aids**: These are substances classified as drugs or hormonal products that may help improve performance. Examples include anabolic steroids, growth hormone, erythropoietin (EPO), and anti-inflammatory drugs (NSAIDs).

- **Physiological Ergogenic Aids**: These are procedures or strategies that may produce a physiological effect resulting in performance enhancement. Examples include blood doping, altitude/hypoxic training, and intermittent hypoxic training.
- **Psychological Ergogenic Aids**: These are strategies or techniques aimed at producing a psychological effect that may help improve performance. Examples include visualization, mental rehearsal, pre-competitive routines, and meditation.
- **Biomechanical Ergogenic Aids**: These are technological items or equipment that may help improve an athlete's energy use, technique, or comfort. Examples include advanced sports equipment, footwear, clothing materials, and engineering techniques.

7.1.2 The Use and Regulation of Ergogenic Aids

Due to the competitive nature of sport, athletes often seek an edge over their opponents by incorporating ergogenic aids into their training and competition schedules. With the increasing availability and commercialization of various aids, it is crucial for athletes to be aware of the efficacy, ethical implications, and potential side effects associated with the use of certain substances and techniques.

Many ergogenic aids fall under WADA's (World Anti-Doping Agency) Prohibited List, meaning their use can lead to sanctions and disqualifications. Athletes at all levels must familiarize themselves with this list, and consult with their coaches, trainers, and nutritionists to ensure that they are not inadvertently utilizing a banned substance or technique.

On the other hand, there is a wide range of legal and ethically accepted ergogenic aids available. The key, however, is determining which are most effective and best suited for an individual athlete's needs. Efficacy can vary greatly depending on the individual, the type of sport involved, the level of training, and the athlete's goals. It is essential to weigh the benefits against the risks, as well as the potential ethical implications of incorporating any ergogenic aid into one's regimen.

7.1.3 Evaluating Ergogenic Aids: The ABCD Framework

When it comes to identifying an effective ergogenic aid, you can utilize the ABCD framework to guide your decision-making:

- **A: Authority** - Determine the credibility of the sources that endorse the ergogenic aid. Reliable sources include scientific studies, professional organizations, and experts within the field of sports nutrition or medicine. Be cautious of anecdotal evidence and promotional material, as they may be biased.
- **B: Benefit** - Assess the potential benefits of the ergogenic aid based on scientific evidence. What is the magnitude of the effect, and how has it been measured? It is crucial to consider the study design, consistency of findings, and whether the findings are applicable to your specific situation.
- **C: Cost** - Consider the financial cost of the ergogenic aid, along with potential time investments and adjustments to your training or lifestyle. Weigh these costs against the potential benefits to determine the overall value.
- **D: Danger** - Evaluate the potential side effects, risks, and dangers associated with the use of the ergogenic aid. Consider any known interactions,

contraindications, and adverse events reported in scientific literature.

Applying the ABCD framework can help athletes, coaches, and trainers make informed decisions about which ergogenic aids may be worth further consideration and use.

In conclusion, ergogenic aids can provide a competitive edge for athletes, as they may enhance physical performance and recovery. It is important for athletes to be aware of the efficacy, ethical implications, and potential side effects associated with using these aids. By conducting thorough research and consulting with professionals, athletes can make informed decisions about incorporating ergogenic aids into their training and competition routines.

7.1 Ergogenic Aids: The Science and Controversy Behind Performance-Enhancing Supplements

Ergogenic aids are a hot topic in the athletic world, with many athletes and coaches swearing by the positive impact that specific supplements and performance-enhancing compounds have on performance. The lure of improved strength, endurance, and recovery can be difficult to resist, and as a result, the sports nutrition industry is booming. However, the use of ergogenic aids is also a source of controversy and debate, with concerns about long-term health consequences, ethical issues, and regulations within professional sports. In this section, we'll dive into the science behind some of the most popular ergogenic aids, weigh their pros and cons, and help you make informed decisions about supplementing your athletic endeavors.

7.1.1 Creatine: Powering Your Muscles for Performance and Adaptation

Creatine is one of the most well-known and well-researched ergogenic aids in the world of sports nutrition. This compound is a natural component of the diet, primarily found in meat and fish, and it plays a crucial role in providing rapid energy to muscles during high-intensity exercise by converting adenosine diphosphate (ADP) back into adenosine triphosphate (ATP). When an athlete supplements with creatine, their muscles are able to store more phosphocreatine, which can extend the duration of high-intensity exercise before fatigue sets in.

Pros: Creatine has well-established benefits for high-intensity, short-duration exercises like lifting weights, sprinting, or jumping. Research has shown that taking 3-5 grams of creatine per day can increase muscle strength, power output, and lean body mass. This popular supplement is also relatively safe when used within the recommended dosages, with few side effects reported.

Cons: While creatine is widely considered to be safe, there have been occasional reports of gastrointestinal discomfort and muscle cramping, especially when taken in larger amounts or without adequate hydration. Additionally, regular creatine supplementation may not always be necessary, as creatine stores in the muscles can become saturated within a few days of beginning supplementation, and will remain elevated for several weeks after ceasing supplementation. Finally, the beneficial effects of creatine are primarily limited to high-intensity, short-duration activities, so endurance athletes and those involved in extended-duration sports may not experience significant performance enhancements from creatine supplementation.

7.1.2 Beta-Alanine: Buffering Your Way to Endurance and Reduced Fatigue

Beta-alanine, a non-essential amino acid, has gained attention in recent years for its potential ergogenic effects, specifically its ability to increase muscle carnosine content. Carnosine acts as a pH buffer within muscles, neutralizing the acidic buildup that occurs during high-intensity exercise and can lead to muscle fatigue. Unfortunately, carnosine can't be efficiently supplemented orally, so researchers have turned to beta-alanine as a way to indirectly boost carnosine levels.

Pros: Studies on beta-alanine supplementation have revealed promising results for athletes participating in high-intensity, intermittent exercises or events lasting between 1 and 10 minutes. Athletes who supplement with 2-5 grams of beta-alanine per day have shown improvements in exercise capacity and reductions in perceived fatigue. Furthermore, combining beta-alanine with other ergogenic aids, such as creatine, may lead to additional performance benefits.

Cons: Despite its potential benefits, beta-alanine is not without drawbacks. Some people will experience a harmless tingling sensation (paresthesia) after consuming larger doses of the supplement, which can be uncomfortable but typically subsides within an hour. More importantly, the research on beta-alanine is currently limited, and the extent of its ergogenic effects on athletic performance is not fully understood. Additionally, beta-alanine may not be effective for all athletes, as its benefits seem to be mostly limited to events that significantly challenge an athlete's anaerobic capacity.

7.1.3 Caffeine: A Time-Tested and Effective Performance Enhancer

Caffeine, a natural stimulant and the world's most widely consumed psychoactive substance, has long been used by athletes to improve performance. Numerous studies have documented the efficacy of caffeine as an ergogenic aid, with benefits that include enhanced muscle endurance, reduced perceived exertion, and improved focus during training and competition.

Pros: The research supporting the ergogenic effects of caffeine on athletic performance is vast, and benefits have been demonstrated for a wide range of sports and activities, including endurance events, intermittent high-intensity sports, and various types of strength training. Dosages of 3-6 milligrams of caffeine per kilogram of body weight have been shown to be effective, and for most individuals, these doses are considered safe.

Cons: While caffeine is both effective and generally safe, it can have negative effects for some individuals. These may include increased heart rate, jitters or nervousness, gastrointestinal distress, and sleep disturbances. Additionally, long-term, habitual use of caffeine can lead to a reduced sensitivity to its effects, which may negate some or all of its ergogenic benefits. Finally, some athletes may need to be cautious with their caffeine intake, as certain sports organizations and events have established upper limits for caffeine concentrations in blood and urine samples.

7.1.4 Nitrate Supplementation: Boosting Oxygen Efficiency for Enhanced Performance

Nitrate supplements have emerged as a popular ergogenic aid in recent years, with potential benefits ranging from enhanced cardiovascular function to improved muscular efficiency during exercise. Nitrate is a compound found naturally in many plant-based foods, such as beets, spinach, and arugula, and is converted in the body to nitric oxide, a potent vasodilator that can improve blood flow and oxygen utilization during exercise.

Pros: One of the most significant advantages of nitrate supplementation, particularly for endurance athletes, is its ability to enhance oxygen efficiency during exercise, meaning athletes are able to maintain a given pace or intensity using less oxygen than they would without supplementation. This can lead to improved exercise economy, endurance capacity, and overall performance. Studies have also shown improvements in muscle contractile efficiency and reduced fatigue with nitrate supplementation.

Cons: While nitrate supplementation may provide benefits for a variety of athletes, the research is still emerging, and the extent of its ergogenic effects may vary between individuals. Additionally, the optimal dosage and timing strategies for nitrate supplementation are not yet clear, with some research suggesting that best results may be obtained by combining dietary sources of nitrate with a supplemental form. Finally, some athletes may experience gastrointestinal side effects or issues with palatability when consuming nitrates as a supplement or in concentrated nitrate-rich foods and beverages.

7.1.5 Legal and Ethical Considerations

While ergogenic aids can offer performance-enhancing benefits, it's essential to consider the legal and ethical implications for athletes involved in competitive sports. Different sports organizations and governing bodies have varying regulations surrounding the use of supplements and performance enhancers, so it's crucial to stay informed about the rules that pertain to your sport and specific competitions. Additionally, some supplements may contain banned substances or be contaminated with prohibited ingredients, so athletes must exercise caution and diligence when selecting products for use.

Lastly, the decision to use ergogenic aids should be viewed through the lens of long-term health, safety, and athletic progress. Over-reliance on supplements may detract from the focus on foundational elements of sports nutrition, such as a well-balanced diet, proper hydration, and an appropriate balance of macronutrients and micronutrients. By staying informed and considering the potential benefits, risks, and ethical implications, athletes can make educated decisions about which ergogenic aids, if any, are appropriate for their unique circumstances and goals.

7.1 The Role of Ergogenic Aids in Athletic Performance

Ergogenic aids can be defined as any external influences or factors that help to enhance or boost an athlete's performance. These may include dietary supplements, medications, sports equipment or specific strategies that are employed to boost an individual's skill, strength, endurance or focus during training sessions and/or competitive events.

A vast array of ergogenic aids is available today, with various claims on their efficacy, safety and legality. Some of the most common ergogenic aids include nutritional supplements such as vitamins, minerals, proteins, and carbohydrates; stimulants, such as caffeine and amphetamines; and anabolic agents, such as testosterone and growth hormone. In this chapter, we will focus on the science behind these supplements and how they relate to athletic performance, with special emphasis on their safety and efficacy.

7.1.1 Nutritional Supplements

Nutritional supplements have become increasingly popular among athletes, as well as the general public. They can help bridge the gap between an athlete's daily nutrient requirements and what they receive through their regular diet. However, it is essential to note that the primary source of nutrients for an athlete should always be a balanced and wholesome diet. Supplements should only be considered when a deficiency exists or when their benefits can be proved by scientific data.

Protein Supplements: Protein is a crucial nutrient for athletes, as it helps in the repair, maintenance, and growth of muscle tissue. Many athletes turn to protein supplements, such as whey and casein proteins, to maximize muscle repair and growth after intense workouts. The efficacy of these supplements depends on their quality and the protein content. It has been found that consuming 20-40 grams of high-quality protein, particularly one with a complete amino acid profile, within 1-2 hours after exercise, maximizes muscle protein synthesis.

Carbohydrate Supplements: Carbohydrates are the primary energy source for athletes during physical activities. During endurance or high-intensity activities, carbohydrate stores, particularly in the form of glycogen, can become depleted. Carbohydrate supplements, such as sports gels or drinks, can help to replenish glycogen stores rapidly and enhance performance during these activities. Research suggests that consuming 30-60 grams of carbohydrates per hour during endurance events has a positive impact on performance.

Vitamins and Minerals: Micronutrient supplementation can also play a role in athletic performance. Specific vitamins and minerals, such as B-complex vitamins, vitamin D, calcium, and iron, are essential for energy production, muscle function, and overall health. Supplementation with these micronutrients may be necessary if an athlete's diet does not provide adequate amounts or absorption is compromised due to specific conditions.

7.1.2 Stimulants and Performance Enhancers

Stimulants can provide short-term enhancements in athletic performance by increasing alertness, cognition, and endurance. Several stimulants are banned or regulated by major sports governing bodies due to potential health risks and ethical concerns.

Caffeine: Caffeine is one of the most widely used and well-studied ergogenic aids among athletes. It works by blocking adenosine receptors, leading to increased arousal, alertness, and focus. Research suggests that caffeine can improve endurance, strength, and power output during exercise. The optimal range for athletes depends on individual sensitivities, but a dosage of 3-6 mg/kg body weight, consumed 30-60 minutes before competition, appears to be most effective.

Amphetamines: These are powerful central nervous system stimulants that increase alertness, concentration, and energy levels. Amphetamines have a well-documented potential for abuse, addiction, and serious health risks. As a result, these substances are banned in competitive sports and should be avoided by athletes at all levels.

7.1.3 Anabolic Agents

Anabolic agents are a class of ergogenic aids designed to boost muscle growth and enhance performance by increasing protein synthesis and reducing muscle breakdown. These substances are typically classified as illegal and are banned in competitive sports due to the potential health risks, ethical concerns, and unfair competitive advantage.

Testosterone and Anabolic Steroids: These synthetic hormones mimic the effects of testosterone, promoting muscle growth, rapid recovery, and increased strength. Unfortunately, the use of anabolic steroids comes with significant side effects, including hormonal imbalances, liver damage, and cardiovascular health risks. They are banned substances in most competitive sports, and their risks outweigh any potential performance gains.

Growth Hormone: Human growth hormone (HGH) is a hormone naturally produced by the pituitary gland. It plays a vital role in overall growth and development, as well as recovery and cellular repair. Athletes have used HGH supplementation to enhance muscle growth, reduce body fat, and speed up recovery. However, HGH use comes with side effects, such as joint pain, fluid retention, and an increased risk for diabetes and heart disease. These risks, coupled with the legality and ethical issues, make HGH supplementation ill-advised for athletes.

In conclusion, ergogenic aids have the potential to improve athletic performance. However, it is essential for athletes to make informed decisions regarding their use. A strong emphasis should be placed on using legal, safe, and scientifically proven aids, in conjunction with a balanced and nutrient-dense diet. Additionally, athletes should work closely with coaches, nutritionists, and medical professionals to create a personalized plan to help them achieve optimal performance in their specific sport.

8. Dietary Considerations for Different Sports: Tailoring Nutrition to Your Goals

8.4 Matching Macronutrients to Your Sport: Balancing Carbohydrates, Proteins, and Fats

When it comes to athletic performance, it's essential to match your macronutrient intake to the specific demands of your sport. By doing so, you will ensure that you are fueling your body with the right balance of carbohydrates, proteins, and fats to optimize your performance and recovery. In this section, we'll explore the ideal macronutrient balance for a variety of sports, including endurance sports, strength-based sports, and team sports, while also providing guidelines for how to adjust your intake based on your individual needs.

8.4.1 Endurance Sports

Endurance sports, such as long-distance running, cycling, and swimming, require a high level of aerobic fitness and the ability to sustain activity for extended periods. As a result, the primary macronutrient athletes in these sports need is carbohydrates.

Carbohydrates

During endurance events, the body relies heavily on carbohydrates for fuel. This is because carbohydrates are the most efficient and readily available source of energy for the working muscles. It is recommended that endurance athletes consume a high-carbohydrate diet, with approximately 60-70% of their total daily calories coming from carbs. This ensures that the body has enough glycogen stores to provide energy for long-duration workouts and races.

Some effective carbohydrate sources for endurance athletes include whole grains, fruits, vegetables, and legumes. It is essential for athletes to prioritize complex carbohydrates over simple sugars, as they provide a more sustainable energy source.

Proteins

While carbohydrates are the primary fuel for endurance athletes, adequate protein intake is also essential to support muscle repair and recovery. It is recommended that endurance athletes consume approximately 1.2-1.4 grams of protein per kilogram of body weight each day. This will help to maintain muscle mass and promote recovery after exercise.

High-quality protein sources for endurance athletes include lean meats, fish, poultry, dairy products, legumes, soy products, and certain grains such as quinoa.

Fats

Endurance athletes should not neglect fat intake, as healthy fats play a crucial role in supporting overall health and providing energy during low-intensity aerobic exercise. Aim for 20-30% of your daily calories from healthy fats, found in sources like nuts, seeds, avocados, and olive oil.

8.4.2 Strength-Based Sports

Strength-based sports include weightlifting, powerlifting, bodybuilding, and gymnastics. In contrast to endurance sports, athletes in these disciplines rely more on anaerobic energy systems and often require more protein for muscle growth and repair.

Carbohydrates

Carbohydrate intake is still essential for strength-based athletes; however, it may be slightly lower than that of endurance athletes. Approximately 45-55% of total daily calories from carbohydrates is appropriate for those participating in strength-based sports. Ingesting a source of quick-digesting carbohydrates before and after resistance training can promote muscle glycogen replenishment and faster recovery.

Proteins

Protein intake is a priority for strength-based athletes, as it's vital for muscle growth and repair. Recommended protein intake for this group ranges from 1.6-2.2 grams per kilogram of body weight each day, depending on the intensity and volume of training.

Quality protein sources for strength-based athletes are similar to those for endurance athletes, with an emphasis on lean meats, fish, poultry, dairy, legumes, and soy products.

Fats

Healthy fats are essential for strength-based athletes, as they support joint health, help absorb fat-soluble vitamins, and provide a long-term energy source. Aim for 25-35% of daily calories from healthy fats, focusing on sources like nuts, seeds, avocados, and olive oil.

8.4.3 Team and Mixed Sports

Team and mixed sports include activities like soccer, basketball, rugby, and volleyball. These sports often require a combination of aerobic and anaerobic energy systems and involve elements of both endurance and strength-based activity.

Carbohydrates

Carbohydrates play a crucial role in fueling both aerobic and anaerobic activity in team and mixed sports. Aim for 50-60% of total daily calories from carbohydrates, prioritizing complex carbs from whole grains, fruits, vegetables, and legumes.

Proteins

Protein is also essential for athletes participating in team and mixed sports to support muscle growth, repair, and recovery. Target 1.4-1.7 grams of protein per kilogram of body weight each day, with an emphasis on high-quality sources.

Fats

As with other athletic disciplines, healthy fats are vital for overall health and providing sustained energy. Aim for 25-35% of daily calories from healthy fats like nuts, seeds, avocados, and olive oil.

8.4.4 Individualizing Your Macronutrient Goals

While the guidelines provided above offer a good starting point, it's important to remember that individual needs can vary. Factors such as body composition, training volume, and personal preferences can all affect the ideal balance of macronutrients for each athlete.

Experiment with different macronutrient ratios to find what works best for you and your sport, and consider consulting with a sports dietitian or nutritionist for personalized guidance.

In conclusion, understanding the unique macronutrient requirements of your sport and individual needs is essential for optimizing performance and recovery. By tailoring your macronutrient intake to align with the demands of your sport and personal health goals, you'll be setting yourself up for athletic success.

8.1 Nutrition Guidelines And Strategies For Various Sports

Different sports require varying amounts of strength, endurance, power, and agility. As such, it is essential to tailor your nutritional strategies and guidelines to suit the specific demands of the sport you are engaged in. In this section, we will outline nutritional considerations and recommendations for several popular sports, including endurance sports, strength and power sports, team sports and aesthetic sports. You will learn how to optimize your diet to improve your performance, reduce the risk of injury, and support your goals.

8.1.1 Endurance Sports (Marathon, Cycling, Triathlon)

Endurance sports place a considerable demand on the body, requiring athletes to maintain prolonged periods of activity. To fuel their bodies effectively, athletes in endurance sports need adequate carbohydrates, proper hydration, and nutrient-dense meals.

- **Carbohydrates:** Carbohydrates are the primary fuel source for endurance athletes. They should form the foundation of your diet, consisting of anywhere from 60-70% of your total calorie intake. Focus on complex carbohydrates such as whole grains, legumes, fruits and vegetables to ensure you're getting adequate fiber and micronutrients.
- **Protein:** Protein is essential for muscle repair and recovery, but endurance athletes should not overload on protein. Aim for 15-20% of your daily calorie intake. Choose lean protein sources like chicken, turkey, fish, legumes, and low-fat dairy.
- **Fat:** Fat is a secondary fuel source for endurance athletes and should make up around 20-25% of your total calorie intake. Choose healthy fats, such as those found in nuts, seeds, avocados, and fatty fish.
- **Hydration:** Staying properly hydrated is crucial for endurance athletes. Aim to consume fluids steadily throughout the day and avoiding large amounts immediately before exercise. Make sure to consider electrolytes in your hydration strategy, especially for longer training sessions and hot weather.
- **Race-day nutrition:** During endurance events, aim to consume 30-60 grams of carbohydrates per hour, preferably through frequent, small snacks. Examples include energy gels, sports drinks, and fruit. This will help maintain your blood glucose levels and provide a steady source of energy.

8.1.2 Strength and Power Sports (Weightlifting, Bodybuilding, Powerlifting)

Athletes in strength and power sports require a diet rich in protein to support muscle growth, repair, and recovery. They should also include carbohydrates for energy and nutrient-dense foods for overall health.

- **Protein:** Protein is crucial for these athletes, making up about 25-35% of their total daily calorie intake. Quality protein sources include lean meats, fish, poultry, eggs, legumes, and dairy products.
- **Carbohydrates:** Carbohydrates constitute 40-55% of daily calories, with a focus on complex carbs like whole grains, fruits, and vegetables. They provide energy for intense training sessions and help restore glycogen levels post-workout.
- **Fat:** The remaining 20-25% of daily calories should come from fat. Emphasize healthy fats from sources such as nuts, seeds, avocado, and olive oil.
- **Caloric surplus:** To build muscle effectively, athletes in strength and power sports require a slight caloric surplus, ideally by 250-500 extra calories per day.
- **Post-workout nutrition:** Consuming adequate carbohydrates and protein is crucial post-workout. Aim for a 31 to 41 carbohydrate to protein ratio, ideally within 30-60 minutes after training. This will aid in muscle repair, recovery, and growth.

8.1.3 Team Sports (Soccer, Basketball, Football)

Team sports typically involve a mix of aerobic and anaerobic activities. Athletes need balanced nutrition to support energy needs, muscle repair, and overall health.

- **Carbohydrates:** Carbohydrates should make up around 50-60% of daily calories, with a focus on complex sources like whole grains, fruits, and vegetables.
- **Protein:** Protein is vital for muscle repair and growth, making up 20-25% of daily calories for team sports athletes. Include lean meats, fish, poultry, eggs, legumes, and dairy in your diet.
- **Fat:** Aim for healthy fats to constitute 20-25% of daily calorie intake, focusing on nuts, seeds, avocado, and olive oil.
- **Pre-game nutrition:** Carbohydrates are crucial for fueling team sports athletes. Have a carbohydrate-rich meal 2-4 hours before a game, along with some protein to support muscle repair and recovery.

8.1.4 Aesthetic Sports (Gymnastics, Dance, Figure Skating)

Aesthetic sports require strength, flexibility, and precision. These athletes need to maintain optimal body weight and composition without sacrificing performance.

- **Nutrient-dense foods:** Choose nutrient-dense foods like whole grains, fruits, vegetables, lean proteins, and healthy fats to ensure you're getting the most nutrition in the least amount of calories.
- **Energy balance:** Sufficient energy intake is essential to support training demands and maintain a healthy body weight. Monitor body composition regularly and adjust your diet accordingly.
- **Carbohydrates:** Aim for carbohydrates to make up around 50-60% of your daily calorie intake, emphasizing complex sources.

- **Protein:** Protein intake should be 15-20% of daily calories, focusing on lean meats, fish, poultry, eggs, legumes, and dairy products.
- **Fat:** Consume healthy fats, making up around 20-25% of your daily calorie intake, from nuts, seeds, avocado, and olive oil.

In conclusion, tailoring your nutrition to your sport, training demands, and performance goals is vital for success, overall health, and injury prevention. Experiment with different nutritional strategies and consult with a sports nutrition expert to find the best approach for your sport and unique needs. Remember, proper nutrition is a key component of any athlete's training and performance plan.

8.1 Sport-Specific Dietary Needs

While the basics of sports nutrition, such as adequate calorie intake, hydration and macronutrient balance, can be applied universally to all athletes, it is crucial to recognize that some sports demand different dietary considerations to optimize performance. This is largely influenced by the variations in the nature of the sports, their energy systems used, and the specifics of their training regimens. In this section, we will delve deeper into how unique athletic goals from various sports can benefit from tailored nutrition strategies.

8.1.1 Endurance Sports

Endurance sports, such as distance running, cycling, swimming, or triathlon, demand sustained submaximal effort for prolonged durations. In these sports, the main fuel sources are carbohydrates and fats, with glycogen being the predominant energy storage form.

Carbohydrates: The foremost dietary priority for endurance athletes is to maximize their glycogen stores. This can be achieved by consistently consuming high-carbohydrate diets (6-10g of carbohydrates per kg body weight per day) and tapering training leading up to competition. Carbohydrate intake during endurance events lasting more than 90 minutes can also prove helpful in sustaining performance.

Fats: While fat adaptation can assist in increasing the metabolic efficiency of fat oxidation, a diet excessively laden with fats may compromise glycogen stores in endurance athletes. Therefore, it is advisable to maintain a balanced diet with moderate fat intake (20-25% of total energy intake). Omega-3 fatty acids, such as those found in fish oil or chia seeds, are anti-inflammatory and can be beneficial for recovery and injury prevention.

Protein: The protein requirements for endurance athletes range between 1.2-1.8 g per kg body weight per day. Consuming protein along with carbohydrate sources after an endurance workout aids in glycogen resynthesis and speeds up recovery.

8.1.2 Power and Strength Sports

Sports like weightlifting, powerlifting, or short-duration, high-intensity activities such as sprints require bursts of strength and power. Unlike endurance athletes, the primary energy system employed in these sports is anaerobic, which relies significantly on the phosphocreatine system.

Carbohydrates: Unlike endurance athletes, power and strength athletes do not heavily rely on carbohydrate oxidation for energy production. However, adequate glycogen stores remain important for fueling anaerobic glycolytic pathways and ensuring a limited supply of glucose is available during high-intensity efforts. Recommended carbohydrate intake falls in the range of 3-5 g per kg body weight per day.

Fats: As these sports are not characterized by extended durations, fat oxidation does not play a central role in energy provision. Therefore, maintaining a diet with moderate fat intake (20-25% of total energy intake) should provide sufficient energy without hindering glycogen stores.

Protein: Adequate protein intake is crucial for strength and power athletes to support muscle hypertrophy and repair. It is recommended they consume 1.6-2.2 g of protein per kg body weight per day as per their training schedules.

8.1.3. Team Sports

Sports such as soccer, basketball, rugby, and hockey encompass aspects of both endurance and power/speed performance with varying energy demands throughout the game. While carbohydrate and glycogen intake is essential, tailored nutrition strategies should also cater to the intermittent high-intensity aspects of these sports.

Carbohydrates: As these sports feature intermittent high-intensity efforts, glycogen stores play a significant role in maintaining performance levels, similar to endurance sports. Carbohydrate intake may be subjected to position-specific energy demands, but generally should range from 5-8 g per kg body weight per day to ensure optimized energy availability for both aerobic and anaerobic energy pathways.

Fats: Optimal fat intake in team sports should mirror endurance sports while ensuring no excessive intake as it may compromise glycogen stores.

Protein: Protein requirements are similar to those of strength and power sports to aid in recovery and adaptation following the varying intensities during the training and performance of team sports.

8.1.4 Flexibility and Skill-Based Sports

Sports like gymnastics, figure skating, or dance, that require significant flexibility, skill, and precision often place athletes at an increased risk of energy deficiencies due to aesthetically driven body composition goals or weight manipulation practices.

Energy Availability: Results-driven weight loss practices can lead to energy deficiencies, compromising athletic performance and health. Adequate energy intake should tailor to individuals' weight management goals at a gradual pace, ensuring a healthy progression.

Macronutrients: Carbohydrates, the predominant source of energy for the central nervous system, are fundamental in these sports to maintain focus, precision, and well-coordinated movements. Protein intake should follow similar recommendations as strength/power sports athletes (1.6-2.2 g per kg body weight per day) due to the strong muscle contractions and eccentric stress involved.

Bone Health: Increased risk of bone stress injuries may arise due to weight loss or energy deficiencies. To counteract bone density issues, athletes should ensure adequate energy availability alongside a sufficient consumption of calcium and vitamin D to promote bone health.

In conclusion, it is crucial to adapt dietary strategies according to the athlete's specific sport, energy requirements, and individual performance goals. Tailoring macronutrient ratios, timing of intake, and specialized supplementation can positively impact performance, recovery, and overall well-being, thereby allowing the athlete to perform at the peak of their potential.

8.1 Sport-Specific Nutritional Needs

Different sports require varying levels of physical and mental demands on an athlete, and as such, different nutrition plans are necessary based on the goals and requirements of each individual athlete. This section will cover various sports and the specific dietary considerations for each discipline. We will look at endurance sports, strength-based sports, team sports, and individual sports.

8.1.1 Endurance Sports

Examples: Long distance running, cycling, swimming, triathlon, rowing, cross-country skiing

Endurance athletes need sustained energy for prolonged exercise, lasting for an hour or more. They require a diet that will help them optimize their energy levels, promote muscle maintenance, and aid in quick recovery.

- Carbohydrates - Carbohydrates are the main source of fuel for endurance athletes. These athletes should focus on high-quality complex carbohydrates with a low to moderate glycemic index. This includes whole grains, fruits, and vegetables. Endurance athletes should aim for 6 to 10 grams of carbohydrates per kilogram of body weight daily.
- Protein - Adequate protein intake is essential for muscle recovery and repair. Endurance athletes should consume 1.2 to 1.4 grams of protein per

kilogram of body weight daily from sources like lean meats, poultry, fish, beans, and dairy.
- Fats - Fats should account for 20 to 35% of an endurance athlete's total calorie intake. Focus on healthy fats like omega-3s found in fatty fish, nuts, seeds, and olive oil.
- Hydration - Staying hydrated is crucial for endurance athletes, as dehydration can lead to decreased performance and increased risk of injury. Always ensure adequate fluid intake before, during, and after training sessions, aiming for approximately 500ml of water per hour of activity, depending on climate and intensity.

8.1.2 Strength-Based Sports

Examples: Weightlifting, powerlifting, bodybuilding, gymnastics, wrestling, judo

Athletes in strength-based sports require a strong focus on muscle growth and repair, power, and explosive strength. Thus, their nutrition plans should hone in on protein intake, fueling their workouts, and providing necessary nutrients for building and maintaining lean muscle mass.

- Carbohydrates - Provide energy to support high-intensity training sessions. Aim for 4 to 7 grams of carbohydrates per kilogram of body weight daily from whole grains, fruits, and vegetables.
- Protein - Adequate protein intake is essential for muscle growth and repair, as well as maintaining muscle mass during fat loss phases. Strength athletes should aim for 1.6 to 2.0 grams of protein per kilogram of body weight daily, focusing on complete protein sources such as lean meats, poultry, fish,

dairy, and plant-based sources like soy, beans, and quinoa.
- Fats - Healthy fats should make up 20 to 35% of total calorie intake. These fats are essential for maintaining good health and hormone production. Include sources like avocados, nuts, seeds, and olive oil in your diet.
- Hydration - As with all athletes, hydration is essential for strength athletes. Be sure to consume enough water throughout the day and especially during and after training sessions.

8.1.3 Team Sports

Examples: Soccer, basketball, hockey, rugby, football

Team sport athletes require a mix of endurance, strength, speed, and agility, which means their nutritional requirements are a balance between those of endurance and strength athletes. They need to fuel their performance throughout a game, as well as recover quickly between games and training sessions.

- Carbohydrates - The primary source of energy for team sport athletes should come from carbohydrates. Aim for 5 to 7 grams of carbohydrates per kilogram of body weight daily from whole grains, fruits, and vegetables.
- Protein - Adequate protein intake is essential for maintaining and repairing muscle tissue. Team sport athletes should consume 1.4 to 1.7 grams of protein per kilogram of body weight daily from lean meats, poultry, fish, dairy, and plant-based sources.
- Fats - Focus on healthy fats to provide approximately 20 to 35% of total calorie intake. This includes sources such as nuts, seeds, avocados, and olive oil.

- Hydration - Staying hydrated is crucial for team sport athletes, as dehydration can lead to decreased performance and increased risk of injury. Be sure to consume enough water throughout the day and especially during training sessions and games.

8.1.4 Individual Sports

Examples: Tennis, golf, track and field, boxing

Individual sport athletes have unique nutritional requirements based on the specific demands of their sport, with some requiring more endurance, while others focus on strength or agility. It is important for athletes in these sports to work closely with a sports nutritionist or dietitian to develop an individualized nutrition plan tailored to their specific needs.

- Carbohydrates - The amount of carbohydrates required depends on the sport and the individual athlete's performance goals. Aim to consume a mix of complex and simple carbohydrates from whole grains, fruits, and vegetables.
- Protein - Protein intake should be tailored to the individual athlete's goals, such as muscle repair, growth, or maintenance. Aim for around 1.2 to 2.0 grams of protein per kilogram of body weight daily from lean meats, poultry, fish, dairy, and plant-based sources.
- Fats - Healthy fats should provide 20 to 35% of total calorie intake, including sources such as nuts, seeds, avocados, and olive oil.
- Hydration - Proper hydration is essential for optimal performance and recovery. Be sure to consume enough water throughout the day and especially during training sessions and competitions.

In conclusion, athletes across various sports should prioritize proper nutrition tailored to their individual needs and training goals to optimize their performance and recovery. By focusing on the appropriate balance of macronutrients and hydration, athletes in all disciplines can fuel their bodies and minds for success.

8.1 Sport-Specific Nutritional Strategies

Each sport has unique demands on the body, and as a result, athletes can benefit from adapting their nutrition to tailor it to their goals. This subsection outlines sport-specific nutritional strategies, helping you to maximize your performance in your chosen sport.

8.1.1 Endurance Sports (Marathon, Triathlon, Cycling)

Endurance sports demand extended periods of physical exertion, challenging the body's ability to maintain energy levels, hydration, and electrolyte balance. A well-planned nutrition strategy is essential for endurance athletes to optimize their performance during training and competition.

- **Carbohydrates**: In endurance sports, carbohydrates are the primary source of fuel for the working muscles. Consuming adequate carbohydrates during the event can prevent muscle glycogen depletion and delay fatigue. Aim for consuming 30-60 grams of carbohydrates per hour during events lasting longer than 90 minutes. Good carbohydrate sources during the event include sports drinks, gels, and energy bars.
- **Protein**: Endurance athletes should include adequate protein in their diet to support recovery, repair, and adaptation of muscles. A general guideline for endurance athletes is to consume 1.2-1.4 grams of

protein per kilogram of body weight daily. Protein-rich foods include lean meats, fish, eggs, dairy, soy products, legumes, and nuts.

- **Fat**: Dietary fat provides essential fatty acids and serves as an additional source of energy during prolonged exercise. Aim for a moderate fat intake (20-35% of daily calories) from healthy sources such as avocados, nuts, seeds, and olive oil.
- **Hydration and Electrolytes**: Proper hydration and electrolyte balance are crucial for endurance athletes to prevent dehydration, muscle cramps, and heat-related illnesses. Regularly consume water or sports drinks during the event, aiming for 500-1000 mL of fluid every hour. In hot and humid conditions, consider increasing fluid intake and seeking shade when possible.

8.1.2 Strength and Power Sports (Weightlifting, Powerlifting, Bodybuilding)

Strength and power athletes primarily rely on the anaerobic energy system, and their nutrition strategies should support the development of lean muscle mass and optimize recovery between training sessions.

- **Protein**: Protein is of utmost importance for strength and power athletes to support muscle growth, repair, and recovery. Aim for a higher daily protein intake of 1.6-2.2 grams per kilogram of body weight, evenly distributed throughout the day. Good protein sources include lean meats, fish, eggs, dairy, soy products, legumes, and nuts.
- **Carbohydrates**: Carbohydrates provide energy necessary for high-intensity training sessions but should be tailored to fit individual goals. For muscle building, consume approximately 5-6 grams of

carbohydrates per kilogram of body weight daily. For fat loss or maintenance, reduce carbohydrate intake to 3-4 grams per kilogram of body weight.
- **Fat**: Aim for a moderate fat intake (20-35% of daily calories) from healthy sources such as avocados, nuts, seeds, and olive oil.
- **Nutrient Timing**: Strength and power athletes can benefit from proper nutrient timing to optimize muscle recovery and adaptation. Consume a combination of carbohydrates and protein (3:1 ratio) within 30 minutes of completing a workout to replenish glycogen stores and support protein synthesis.

8.1.3 Team Sports (Basketball, Soccer, Hockey)

Team sport athletes require a versatile approach to nutrition that promotes energy for both aerobic and anaerobic capacities, supports muscle recovery between games, and optimizes cognitive function during play.

- **Carbohydrates**: Carbohydrates are essential for maintaining energy levels and preventing muscle glycogen depletion during training and competitions. Aim for consuming 5-7 grams of carbohydrates per kilogram of body weight daily. Prioritize high-quality carbohydrate sources, such as whole grains, fruits, and vegetables.
- **Protein**: Include 1.4-1.7 grams of protein per kilogram of body weight daily to support muscle repair and recovery. Opt for protein-rich foods, like lean meats, fish, eggs, dairy, soy products, legumes, and nuts.
- **Fat**: Aim for a moderate fat intake (20-35% of daily calories) from healthy sources such as avocados, nuts, seeds, and olive oil.
- **Hydration and Electrolytes**: Team sports athletes should prioritize hydration, as fluid losses can

negatively impact performance and cognitive function. Monitor urine color and aim for a pale yellow hue, indicating adequate hydration. Consume water or sports drinks during games or practices, depending on individual sweat rates and sports drink preferences.

- **Caffeine**: Caffeine has been shown to enhance cognitive function, alertness, and reaction time, which can be beneficial for team sport athletes. Consider consuming 3-6 mg/kg of caffeine 30-60 minutes before training or competitions.

8.1.4 Gymnastics, Figure Skating, and Dance

Aesthetic sports, such as gymnastics, figure skating, and dance, require a balance of strength, power, and flexibility. Athletes often have weight-related concerns due to the strong impact of body composition on performance.

- **Energy Intake**: Meeting energy needs is crucial for athletes in aesthetic sports to maintain proper health, reduce injury risk, and optimize performance. Dieticians recommend calculating individual energy requirements based on factors such as body size, gender, age, and training workload. Consult with a sports nutrition professional to determine an appropriate energy intake.
- **Macronutrient Ratios**: Athletes in aesthetic sports should prioritize a balanced diet with sufficient macronutrients, to support performance and overall health. Recommended daily intake includes 1.2-1.7 grams of protein per kilogram of body weight, 3-5 grams of carbohydrates per kilogram of body weight, and 20-35% of total calories from healthy fats.
- **Bone Health**: Adequate intake of calcium and vitamin D is essential for bone health in aesthetic sport

athletes, who often have high levels of impact on their bones and joints. Include calcium-rich foods such as dairy products, leafy greens, and fortified foods in the daily diet, and spend time outdoors to promote natural vitamin D production.

- **Mental Health and Body Image**: Aesthetic sport athletes may face higher pressures regarding body image, potentially leading to disordered eating and a negative relationship with food. Athletes should focus on consuming nutrient-dense foods to fuel their body and support performance, rather than dieting to achieve a specific body weight or shape.

Each sport demands a unique approach to nutrition, providing athletes the opportunity to tailor their diet to optimize performance and achieve their goals. Working with a professional sports nutritionist can further refine specific nutritional strategies and address any challenges faced in meeting competition, performance, or training requirements. Ultimately, a well-designed sport-specific nutritional plan can promote peak performance and support overall health in athletes.

9. Managing Weight and Body Composition: Strategies for Healthy Performance

9.1 Understanding the Need for Weight Management and Optimal Body Composition

Whether you're a professional athlete, a weekend warrior, or someone who enjoys staying active, understanding how to manage your weight and optimize your body composition is crucial to achieving peak performance levels. In this section, we will discuss why different athletes need different body compositions, how to assess your current body composition state, the factors influencing body composition, and strategies to achieve a healthy and optimal weight for your sport.

9.1.1 Importance of Weight Management and Optimal Body Composition in Athletes

In sports and athletic performance, body composition plays a crucial role. It refers to the body's proportions of fat, muscle, bone, and water. The amount of each component varies depending on the individual and their specific athletic goals. In general, a lower body fat percentage and higher muscle mass are favorable for optimal athletic performance. Optimal body composition can provide various benefits such as:

- Improved power-to-weight ratio which can help in various sports like running, cycling, and gymnastics.
- Increased strength, endurance, and agility.
- Reduced risk of injury, since excess fat can place additional stress on joints.
- Enhanced recovery and response to training, as a higher lean body mass is better equipped to repair and regenerate.
- Ideal body composition also has a psychological benefit as it increases confidence and self-esteem in athletes.

It is essential to remember that there is no single "perfect" body composition for all athletes. Different athletes will require different body fat levels, muscular development, and overall body mass, depending on the sports they play and the specific demands of their events. For instance, marathon runners will generally have a lower body fat percentage compared to powerlifters, while a basketball player would require a balance between muscle mass and agility for optimal performance.

9.1.2 Assessing Body Composition

Before implementing any strategies to manage your weight and body composition, it is crucial to establish your current baseline. There are several methods to measure and track body composition, some of which include:

1. **Skinfold Calipers**: A common and relatively affordable method, where the thickness of subcutaneous fat is measured using calipers at specific sites on the body.
2. **Bioelectrical Impedance Analysis (BIA)**: A device that measures the rate at which a weak electrical current travels through the body. Fat, muscle, and

water have different resistance levels, which can be used to estimate body composition.
3. **Dual-Energy X-Ray Absorptiometry (DEXA)**: A more advanced and accurate method, which scans the entire body to provide detailed information on fat, muscle, and bone distribution.
4. **Bod Pod**: An air displacement method that uses pressure changes in a sealed chamber to determine body density, which can then be used to estimate body composition.

Regular assessment of body composition can help you determine if you are making the desired progress towards your athletic goals, and also provides a more complete picture of body changes compared to just tracking weight on a scale.

9.1.3 Factors Influencing Body Composition

Several factors can impact an athlete's body composition, and understanding these can assist in implementing effective weight and body composition management strategies. Some key factors include:

1. **Genetics**: Each individual inherits a unique set of genes that can influence how their body stores fat and builds muscle.
2. **Age**: As we age, our metabolism slows down, causing shifts in body composition.
3. **Gender**: Males tend to have a higher muscle mass, whereas females generally have a higher fat mass due to hormonal differences.
4. **Diet**: The quantity, quality, and timing of food intake play an essential role in determining body composition.

5. **Physical Activity**: The type, intensity, frequency, and duration of exercise can influence how the body utilizes energy, stores fat, and builds muscle.
6. **Sleep**: Adequate sleep is crucial for regulating hormones and promoting tissue growth, repair, and recovery.

9.1.4 Strategies for Achieving Healthy Weight and Optimal Body Composition

Now that you have an understanding of the importance of body composition and the factors influencing it, here are some strategies to help you manage your weight and achieve optimal body composition for your sports performance:

1. **Maintain a Balanced Diet**: Ensure that your diet comprises an appropriate mix of carbohydrates, proteins, and fats, catering to your specific sports demands and athletic goals.
2. **Monitor Caloric Intake**: Use tools such as calorie counters and food journals to track your daily energy intake and ensure that you're consuming an appropriate number of calories to support your training and maintain a healthy weight.
3. **Periodization of Nutrition**: Plan your diet to match your training phases, adjusting your caloric intake and macronutrient ratios to optimize fueling, recovery, and adaptation.
4. **Optimize Protein Intake**: Consuming an appropriate amount of protein across the day and during various times (pre- and post-exercise) can help support muscle repair, growth, and maintenance.
5. **Incorporate Resistance Training**: Include strength and resistance training in your exercise routine to

build lean muscle mass and promote favorable changes in body composition.

6. **Prioritize Recovery**: Ensure adequate rest, sleep, and stress management to support the body's natural processes of repair, regeneration, and hormonal balance.
7. **Smart Cardio Training**: Use different intensities, durations, and types of aerobic exercise to help burn excess body fat without compromising muscle mass.

Achieving optimal body composition for your sport is a multifaceted approach that requires consistent efforts in both nutrition and training. Always consult with a registered dietitian and a professional coach to develop a personalized plan that satisfies your specific needs and ensures long-term success in your athletic endeavors.

9.1 Monitoring Your Weight and Body Composition: The Importance of Consistency and Accuracy

9.1.1 Understanding Body Composition

Body composition refers to the percentage of body weight that is made up of fat mass and fat-free mass (lean body mass). Lean body mass includes muscle, bones, organs, and water, while fat mass refers to both essential fat (needed for vital body functions) and stored fat (used for insulation, cushioning, and energy storage). Knowing your body composition is essential for athletes because it helps identify the most suitable training and nutrition strategies, as well as for monitoring progress and evaluating the effectiveness of these strategies.

9.1.2 Monitoring Tools and Techniques

There are several techniques available to measure body composition, each with varying levels of accuracy, practicality, and cost. Some of the most common methods used are:

- *Bioelectrical impedance analysis (BIA)*: This technique sends a low-level electrical current through the body and measures the resistance (impedance) of body tissues. As fat mass and lean body mass conduct electricity differently, this method provides an estimate of body composition.
- *Skinfold caliper tests*: In this method, the thickness of skinfolds at specific body areas is measured using calipers. These measurements are then used to estimate body fat percentage based on equations that take account of age, gender, and ethnicity.
- *Dual-energy x-ray absorptiometry (DXA)*: This technique involves passing a low-dose x-ray beam through the body to determine bone density, muscle mass, and fat mass. Although accurate, DXA is relatively expensive and time-consuming compared to other methods.
- *Air displacement plethysmography (Bod Pod)*: The Bod Pod is a specialized chamber that measures body volume by monitoring pressure changes resulting from the displacement of air. By combining this data with body weight, body composition can be estimated.
- *Hydrostatic weighing (underwater weighing)*: This technique involves immersing the individual in water to determine body volume, which is then used to calculate body density and composition. Although accurate, hydrostatic weighing can be impractical and uncomfortable for some individuals.

Whatever method you choose, it is essential to maintain consistency throughout your monitoring process. This means measuring your body composition under similar conditions, such as the same time of day, hydration status, and pre-assessment routine. This will help you track changes accurately while minimizing the potential for any discrepancies.

9.1.3 Interpreting Body Composition Results

When analyzing your body composition measurements, it's essential to understand that there are no universally "ideal" body fat percentages for all athletes. The optimal body composition varies depending on factors like genetics, sport, training history, and personal preference. However, general recommendations can serve as a starting point.

For male athletes, a body fat percentage of 6-24% is typically considered acceptable, while female athletes may aim for around 16-30%. Keep in mind that achieving a body fat percentage on the lower end of these ranges can improve performance for some sports (like distance running or cycling), but may not be necessary or beneficial for others (such as strength-based sports). Additionally, maintaining a body fat percentage that is too low for an extended period can negatively impact hormonal balance, immune function, and overall health.

9.1.4 Implementing Changes and Tracking Progress

It's essential to remember that the key to achieving sustainable changes in body composition is to prioritize training and nutrition strategies that support long-term health and performance. Focus on adjusting your energy intake, macronutrient balance, meal timing, and training stimulus to promote the desired adaptations (whether that is increasing lean mass or decreasing body fat).

To track progress in terms of body weight and composition, it can be helpful to measure on a consistent schedule. Weekly measurements can provide valuable insights into the effectiveness of your strategies, as well as identify any potential issues that may require further attention. Furthermore, tracking your body composition can also be motivating and provide reinforcement for your effort and commitment to your athletic goals.

By managing your weight and body composition effectively, you can optimize your performance, reduce the risk of injury, and promote overall health and well-being throughout your training and competitive seasons. Remember that achieving optimal body composition is a dynamic process that requires consistent monitoring, evaluation, and adjustments to support your athletic endeavors.

9.1 The Importance of Weight Management in Athletic Performance

Regardless of the sport, body composition and weight management play a major role in an athlete's performance. Athletes, particularly those in sports that require speed, strength, and agility, must maintain the ideal balance between muscle mass, body fat percentage, and total body weight. By optimizing weight management, athletes can:

- Enhance athletic performance in terms of speed, power, and stamina.
- Decrease the risk of injuries, both acute and chronic.
- Improve body awareness and self-regulation in terms of nutritional and training demands.

- Promote long-term health and longevity as an athlete.

9.1.1 Determining Optimal Body Composition

An athlete's ideal body composition is determined by their unique individual needs and sport-specific demands. However, it is essential to maintain healthy body fat levels while maximizing lean mass, which includes muscles, bones, and connective tissues.

Factors that can impact optimal body composition for athletes include:

- **Sport and position**: The body composition requirements for an endurance runner will vastly differ from those of a football lineman. It is essential to consider the unique physical demands of your sport and position and adjust your body composition goals accordingly.
- **Genetics**: Some athletes may naturally have a higher body fat percentage or more muscle mass than others, with genetics playing a significant role in determining these factors.
- **Age**: As athletes age, the distribution of fat and muscle tissue can change, potentially requiring adjustments in body composition goals.
- **Injury and illness**: Injuries and illnesses can significantly impact an athlete's body composition, requiring adjustments to training, nutrition, and recovery plans.

9.1.2 Assessing and Monitoring Weight and Body Composition

Athletes can use several methods to assess and monitor body composition regularly to track progress and make necessary adjustments to their nutrition, training, and recovery plans. Some of the most commonly used methods include:

- **Skinfold measurements**: Skinfold calipers are used to measure the thickness of subcutaneous fat layers, which are then used to estimate overall body mass composition. While this method can be cost-effective and reliable, it requires a skilled professional to accurately measure and interpret results.
- **Bioelectrical impedance**: This technique measures the resistance of body tissues to a small electrical current, providing an estimate of body fat percentage. While portable and straightforward to use, results can be influenced by several factors, including hydration levels and recent food intake.
- **Dual-energy X-ray absorptiometry (DEXA)**: DEXA scans use low-dose X-rays to provide an accurate and detailed assessment of body composition, including data on muscle mass, body fat distribution, and bone density. While DEXA scans are considered the gold standard for body composition analysis, they can be expensive and less accessible for some athletes.

9.1.3 Creating a Weight Management Strategy

With an understanding of the importance of weight management and a method for monitoring body composition, athletes can begin to develop a comprehensive strategy for managing weight and body composition. The following elements are integral components of an effective weight management strategy:

1. **Balanced nutrition**: Consuming the right mix of macronutrients (proteins, carbohydrates, and fats) and micronutrients (vitamins and minerals) is crucial for maintaining optimal body composition. Monitor your caloric intake and make adjustments as necessary to ensure that you are fueling your body appropriately for your sport's demands and goals.
2. **Exercise programming**: Consistently engaging in a balanced exercise program that combines resistance training, cardiovascular exercise, and flexibility is crucial for managing body composition. Tailor your training regimen to target key areas of muscle development and fat reduction based on your sport-specific demands.
3. **Recovery and stress management**: Pay attention to your body's need for rest and recovery, and be mindful of stressors that could hinder your progress. Implement strategies to prioritize sleep, manage stress, and engage in active recovery activities such as massage, foam rolling, and stretching.
4. **Seek guidance**: Work with professionals, including coaches, trainers, and sports nutritionists, to develop and constantly adjust your weight management strategy based on your unique needs and goals. Regular monitoring and feedback are crucial for optimizing your performance.

Conclusion

Learning to manage your weight and body composition is an essential skill in achieving and maintaining peak athletic performance. By understanding the factors that contribute to optimal body composition, monitoring progress, and implementing a personalized weight management strategy, athletes can set themselves up for long-term success in their sport.

9.2. The Importance of a Balanced Diet and Planning Meals

A balanced diet plays a pivotal role in maintaining the desired weight and body composition needed for peak athletic performance. Optimal nutrition not only fuels workouts but also aids in recovery and reduces the risk of injuries. To strike the perfect balance in the diet, athletes must consider their daily caloric needs, the quality of the nutrients ingested, and appropriate meal-timing strategies.

9.2.1. Caloric Needs

Energy intake must be aligned with the energy expended during daily activities and workouts. A caloric surplus will lead to weight gain, while a deficit will result in weight loss. For athletes, either scenario could hinder performance.

Start by determining the Basal Metabolic Rate (BMR), which is the number of calories your body needs to maintain its weight without activity. Then, factor in your daily activities and training sessions to calculate your Total Daily Energy Expenditure (TDEE). Meeting the TDEE through dietary intake will maintain the body weight, while a surplus or deficit of 10-20% will lead to controlled weight gain or loss, respectively. The ideal caloric intake depends on factors such as age, gender, body composition, and performance goals.

9.2.2. Quality of Nutrients

The quality of nutrients is as important as the quantity. A balanced diet must provide a sufficient amount of carbohydrates, proteins, fats, vitamins, and minerals. Each of these macronutrients plays a crucial role in achieving and maintaining optimal athletic performance.

- **Carbohydrates**: As the primary source of energy, carbs are essential for both endurance and high-intensity sports. Consuming carbohydrates should account for about 45-65% of an athlete's caloric intake. Prioritize consuming complex carbs such as whole grains, fruits, and vegetables over simple sugars found in refined or processed foods.
- **Proteins**: Protein is vital for muscle growth, maintenance, and repair, as well as for optimal immune function. About 10-35% of an athlete's daily caloric intake should come from protein. Sources of protein include lean meats, dairy products, and plant-based options like beans and legumes.
- **Fats**: Fats are necessary for energy production, vitamin absorption, and hormone production. Healthy fats, which should account for 20-35% of daily caloric intake, can be found in nuts, seeds, avocados, olive oil, and fatty fish.
- **Vitamins and Minerals**: Micronutrients have numerous vital functions ranging from maintaining strong bones, producing energy, and ensuring a healthy immune system. Focus on eating a varied and nutrient-dense diet to provide your body with the required vitamins and minerals, and consider supplementation only in case of deficiencies.

9.2.3. Meal Planning and Timing

Planning and organizing meals can help athletes adhere to their nutrition requirements more effectively. Regular meal patterns and consistency prevent skipping meals, overeating, or indulging in high-calorie, nutrient-poor foods.

- **Breakfast**: Never skip breakfast! It kickstarts metabolism and helps restore glycogen stores depleted during sleep. A high-quality breakfast is the foundation of the day and should include complex carbs, protein, and healthy fats.
- **Snacks**: Plan 2-3 snacks throughout the day to maintain energy levels and prevent hunger spikes. Reach for nutrient-dense options like nuts, yogurt, fruit, or a protein shake.
- **Pre-workout**: Consuming a meal or snack 1-4 hours before training helps fuel the session. A mix of carbohydrates and protein can optimize energy levels without causing gastrointestinal discomfort during exercise.
- **Post-workout**: Your recovery meal should be consumed within 30 minutes to 2 hours after completing a workout. It should include a mix of carbohydrates and proteins to replenish glycogen stores and repair muscle tissues.
- **Dinner**: A balanced dinner should contain carbohydrates, proteins, and healthy fats. The emphasis should be on lean proteins and a generous portion of colorful vegetables to provide essential micronutrients.

Tracking meals using food diaries or nutrition apps can help athletes ensure they receive the right balance of macronutrients, meeting their caloric needs, and enhancing overall performance. By following a well-thought-out plan and making necessary adjustments as training schedules change, athletes can achieve and maintain their ideal weight and body composition for optimal performance.

9.3 Creating a Balanced Meal Plan for Improved Athletic Performance

Understanding the importance and role of nutrition in athletic performance is essential for managing your weight and improving your body composition. Creating a balanced meal plan that suits your individual needs, sports requirements, and preferences will optimize your ability to perform and recover. Here, we outline some strategies to help you plan a healthy, balanced, and performance-enhancing meal plan.

9.3.1 Assessing Your Nutritional Requirements

Before creating a meal plan, it's essential to assess your individual nutritional requirements based on your:

1. Age
2. Gender
3. Body size and composition
4. Training volume, intensity, and type
5. Personal goals (e.g., weight loss, performance, muscle gain)

To create a personalized meal plan, first, use the following guidelines to determine your daily caloric requirements:

- **Resting energy expenditure (REE)** – This is the amount of energy required to maintain your basic bodily functions at rest, such as breathing, maintaining body temperature, and cell production. It's mainly determined by your age, gender, and body size.
- **Physical activity level (PAL)** – This measures the additional calories burned through physical activity, including sports, exercise, and daily activities. PAL varies greatly depending on the type, duration, and intensity of your training.

- **Total energy expenditure (TEE)** – This is the total amount of calories you need to meet your energy demands, including both REE and PAL.

Next, determine your macronutrient distribution, which is the proportion of carbohydrates, proteins, and fats in your diet. The following guidelines generally apply to athletes:

- Carbohydrates: 45-65% of total daily calorie intake
- Proteins: 10-35% of total daily calorie intake
- Fats: 20-35% of total daily calorie intake

9.3.2 Building a Balanced Meal Plan

A meal plan that promotes athletic performance, weight management, and overall health should include an appropriate balance of macronutrients, emphasizing nutrient-dense and minimally processed foods. Here are some tips for building a balanced meal plan:

Carbohydrates

As the body's primary fuel source, carbohydrates should be at the foundation of an athlete's diet. Focus on consuming complex carbohydrates from whole grains (e.g., brown rice, whole wheat pasta, quinoa, barley), starchy vegetables (e.g., sweet potatoes, pumpkin, peas), and legumes (e.g., black beans, lentils, chickpeas). Consumption of fibrous carbs such as leafy greens, cruciferous vegetables (e.g., broccoli, cauliflower), and colorful fruits (e.g., berries, oranges, kiwifruit) will provide vitamins, minerals, and antioxidants to complement your performance.

Proteins

Include high-quality protein sources in each meal and snack to support muscle repair and growth, immune function, and overall health. Excellent protein sources include lean meat, poultry, fish, eggs, dairy (e.g., Greek yogurt, cottage cheese), and plant-based options like tofu, tempeh, edamame, and beans. Aim for at least 1.2-2.0 grams of protein per kilogram of body weight daily, depending on your sport and training intensity.

Fats

Choose healthy fats, such as monounsaturated and omega-3 fatty acids, to support your energy needs, cell and hormone development, and overall health. Prioritize sources like avocados, nuts, seeds, fatty fish (e.g., salmon, mackerel), and plant-based oils like olive, avocado, or flaxseed oil. Limit the consumption of saturated fats from processed and fried foods, as they can lead to weight gain and increased health risks.

9.3.3 Timing and Portions

In addition to balancing macronutrients, optimizing meal and snack timing is crucial for fueling your workouts, recovery, and overall performance. Consider the following strategies:

- **Pre-workout**: Eat a light meal or snack containing carbohydrates and protein 1-3 hours before exercising.
- **During workout**: For prolonged exercise (90 minutes or more), consume carbohydrate-rich snacks or sports drinks to maintain energy.
- **Post-workout**: Consume a recovery meal or snack containing carbohydrates and protein within 1-2 hours

of finishing a workout, with specific recommendations varying based on the intensity.

Be mindful of portion sizes, and adjust them to accommodate your daily caloric and macronutrient goals. Use measuring tools like measuring cups, nutrition scales, or hand-based portion guidelines to ensure accurate portion sizes.

9.3.4 Hydration

Proper hydration significantly impacts athletic performance, affecting your heart rate, body temperature regulation, and muscular function. Maintain adequate fluid intake throughout the day, consuming water, coconut water, milk, and unsweetened beverages. Aim to consume at least half of your body weight (in pounds) in fluid ounces daily, with additional fluid intake during and after exercise.

9.3.5 Supplements

While a balanced, whole-foods-based diet should always be the foundation, certain supplements may further support your performance and nutritional goals. Consult with a certified sports dietitian to determine if any supplements are suitable for your specific needs and performance goals.

Remember, a personalized meal plan should evolve with your training, goals, and lifestyle. Be prepared to adjust your meal plan as necessary, and discuss any concerns or questions with a sports dietitian.

Creating a balanced meal plan that prioritizes nutrient-dense foods and proper timing while meeting your individual nutritional requirements is crucial for optimizing your weight management, body composition, and athletic performance. By understanding the fundamental components of a healthy, performance-focused meal plan, you can fuel your body, maximize your potential and achieve your goals.

10. The Mindful Athlete: Understanding Eating Disorders and Body Image in Sports

Eating Disorders: Types, Symptoms, and Causes for Athletes

10.1 Types of Eating Disorders

It's important to understand the various types of eating disorders and to recognize their symptoms. Not only will this help athletes determine if they might be struggling with one, but it will also enable coaches, parents, and teammates to identify potential issues and provide support. Here are the main types of eating disorders that may affect athletes:

1. **Anorexia Nervosa**: This extreme fear of gaining weight can lead to severe calorie restriction, sometimes resulting in potentially life-threatening weight loss. Athletes with anorexia often have a distorted body image, believing that they are much larger or heavier than they actually are.
2. **Bulimia Nervosa**: Bulimia is characterized by recurrent episodes of binge eating, during which the person consumes an unusually large amount of food in a short time frame. This is followed by purging behaviors-like self-induced vomiting, misuse of laxatives, or excessive exercise-to compensate for the excessive caloric intake.

3. **Binge Eating Disorder**: Similar to bulimia, individuals with binge eating disorder may exhibit periods of uncontrollable overeating. However, they do not engage in purging behaviors. Instead, they often feel intense feelings of guilt and shame about their eating habits.
4. **Orthorexia**: While not officially recognized as an eating disorder, orthorexia is described as an unhealthy obsession with "healthy" or "clean" eating. These behaviors may not initially start as harmful, but progressively become severe and negatively impact an individual's physical, mental, and emotional wellbeing.
5. **Female Athlete Triad** (now called Relative Energy Deficiency in Sports or RED-S): A syndrome affecting female athletes, which includes three interrelated components: low energy availability (with or without disordered eating), menstrual dysfunction, and decreased bone mineral density. Athletes with RED-S may experience amenorrhea, decreased athletic performance, and an increased risk of injury.

10.2 Symptoms of Eating Disorders

It's crucial for athletes, coaches, and parents to be familiar with the warning signs of eating disorders, helping them identify potential issues in themselves or their peers. Here are some common symptoms of eating disorders in athletes:

1. **Physical Symptoms**:
   - Excessive weight loss or gain
   - Fainting or dizziness
   - Pale or dry skin
   - Stomach cramps or other gastrointestinal complaints
   - Swelling in the hands and feet

       ○ Dental problems, tooth decay or erosion
       ○ Low body temperature
       ○ Dehydration
       ○ Loss of muscle mass
       ○ Irregular menstruation or amenorrhea

2. **Behavioral Symptoms**:
   - Obsessive calorie counting or measuring of food portions
   - Frequency of food consumption or secretive eating habits
   - Overexercising or exercising despite injury or sickness
   - Wearing baggy clothes to hide weight loss or camouflage their body
   - Becoming socially withdrawn or avoiding social situations involving food
   - Frequent negative comments about their body, size, or appearance
   - Setting overly restrictive rules about food choices or rituals around eating
   - Increased use of dietary supplements, diuretics or laxatives
   - Frequent bathroom visits immediately after eating

3. **Emotional Symptoms**:
   - Intense fear of weight gain or obesity
   - Decreased interest and overall performance in their sports
   - Irritability, mood swings or depression
   - Anxiety around meal times or eating in public
   - Low self-esteem or body dissatisfaction
   - Feelings of guilt or shame about eating
   - Perfectionism, especially when it comes to diet or exercise

10.3 Causes of Eating Disorders in Athletes

There isn't one single cause for an eating disorder; rather, a combination of genetic, environmental, and psychological factors contributes to the development of these conditions. Here are some common factors that make athletes more vulnerable to eating disorders:

1. **Pressure to Perform**: Many sports emphasize weight or body size as being essential to the individual's performance. Consequently, athletes may engage in disordered eating behaviors to maintain a perceived "ideal" body for their sport.
2. **Perfectionism**: Athletes often have high expectations for themselves and their performance, with a desire to excel in their sport. This perfectionism can spill over into their eating habits and self-image, increasing the risk of developing an eating disorder.
3. **Peer and Coach Influence**: Athletes are sometimes pressured by coaches, teammates, or peers to conform to a specific body type or to manage their weight aggressively. This pressure could lead to unhealthy dieting habits, and eventually, disordered eating.
4. **Genetics and Family History**: Eating disorders tend to run in families, and some individuals may have a genetic predisposition to these conditions. Additionally, if an athlete grows up in an environment where others have eating disorders, they may be more likely to develop one themselves.
5. **Media Portrayal**: The media's portrayal of an "ideal" athletic body can contribute to dissatisfaction with one's body. Exposure to images promoting leanness and muscularity can lead athletes to feel inadequate, driving them to try and conform to this unrealistic ideal.

In conclusion, understanding the types, symptoms, and causes of eating disorders among athletes is critical to maintaining their physical and mental health. Athletes, parents, and coaches must be educated on the signs of these disorders and the factors that contribute to their development. This knowledge helps cultivate an environment of support and promotes healthy habits in the world of sports.

10.1 Recognizing Eating Disorders and Body Image Issues in Athletes

Eating disorders and body image issues are prevalent in the world of sports, affecting both elite and recreational athletes. A negative body image and the desire to attain an unrealistic perfect body can lead to severe consequences, including the development of disordered eating behaviors or full-blown eating disorders. In this section, we'll discuss the various types of eating disorders commonly found in athletes, the role of sports culture in their development, and the importance of early intervention and support.

10.1.1 Types of Eating Disorders

Eating disorders are mental health conditions that involve severe disturbances in eating behavior, leading to physical and emotional consequences. The most common eating disorders in athletes include:

1. **Anorexia Nervosa**: characterized by an intense fear of gaining weight, distorted body image, and a severe restriction of food intake, leading to extreme weight loss and severe health complications.
2. **Bulimia Nervosa**: involves repeated episodes of binge eating followed by compensatory behaviors such as self-induced vomiting, excessive exercise,

and/or the misuse of laxatives and diuretics to prevent
weight gain.
3. **Binge Eating Disorder**: recurrent episodes of
consuming large amounts of food, accompanied by
feelings of a loss of control over eating and significant
amounts of distress. Binge eating episodes are not
followed by compensatory behaviors, making the
disorder distinct from bulimia nervosa.
4. **Orthorexia Nervosa**: an extreme fixation on eating
"clean" or "healthy" that becomes psychologically
distressing and interferes with healthy eating, social
functioning, and self-worth.
5. **Other specified feeding and eating disorders
(OSFED)**: do not meet the full diagnostic criteria for
any other specific eating disorder but still cause
significant distress or impairment in daily life.

10.1.2 Sports Culture and Eating Disorders

Several factors contribute to the development and
perpetuation of eating disorders in athletes, including
societal beauty standards, performance expectations, and
the culture of the sports world. Factors specific to athletes
include:

- **Weight-sensitive sports**: in some sports, such as
gymnastics, figure skating, distance running, and
wrestling, there is a perception that success is reliant
upon a lean and light body. This belief can foster the
development of disordered eating behaviors or full-
blown eating disorders as athletes strive to achieve
an ideal body for their sport.
- **Performance pressure**: Athletes face immense
pressure to perform at their peak capacity in
competition, training, and practice. These
expectations lead to a desire to control body weight

and composition, believing it will lead to improved performance.

- **Coaching techniques**: Some coaches may unknowingly contribute to the development of eating disorders by emphasizing the importance of weight management for performance. Additionally, athletes might misinterpret coaches' comments about weight or specific body parts, internalizing them as negative self-evaluations.
- **Comparison and competition**: Athletes often compare themselves to their teammates and competitors in terms of body size, shape, and muscularity. This constant comparison may lead to feelings of inferiority and a desire to engage in disordered eating behaviors to "keep up" with their peers or gain a competitive edge.

10.1.3 The Importance of Early Intervention and Support

Early intervention is crucial in preventing the progression of disordered eating or eating disorders in athletes. The following steps can help athletes, coaches, and support personnel in identifying and addressing these issues:

1. **Education**: Learn about the signs and symptoms of disordered eating and eating disorders. Understand the risk factors and consequences of these conditions for athletes. Stay informed about the latest research and best practices for promoting a positive body image and healthy eating habits.
2. **Screening**: Implement regular screening for disordered eating and eating disorders in athletes. This can include self-report questionnaires, clinical interviews, and multi-disciplinary assessments involving nutritionists and mental health professionals.

3. **Communication**: Encourage open dialogue about body image and eating habits within sports teams and organizations. Address concerns or behaviors promptly and without judgment. Normalize the conversation surrounding mental health and help-seeking in athletes.
4. **Support**: Provide resources and access to qualified professionals, including sports nutritionists, therapists, and medical professionals, who can support athletes in navigating these issues. Create a supportive and inclusive sports environment that prioritizes health, well-being, and self-compassion.
5. **Prevention**: Develop and implement targeted prevention programs and strategies that foster a balanced approach to nutrition, athletic training, and body image in sports. Encourage a holistic approach to athletic performance emphasizing overall health, not solely focused on body size or weight.

Eating disorders and body image issues in athletes are complex and multifaceted problems. By understanding the different types of eating disorders, recognizing the impact of sports culture on these conditions, and emphasizing early intervention and support, coaches, athletes, and support personnel can work together to create a healthy and inclusive environment for all competitors. Remember that a healthy, well-nourished athlete is the most effective athlete!

Eating Disorders, Body Image, and Athletic Performance

Eating disorders are serious psychological conditions, and unfortunately, they are all too common among the athletic community. Athletes typically face a unique set of challenges that may contribute to the development of eating disorders, including pressure to maintain a lean physique, over-emphasis on weight and performance, and exposure to highly competitive environments. Understanding the nature of eating disorders and the role that body image concerns play in their development is crucial to promoting optimal mental and physical health among athletes. In this chapter, we will dive deep into the most common eating disorders within the sports world, the dangerous consequences these disorders can have on athletic performance, and strategies to prevent and treat body image concerns and disordered eating.

Recognizing Eating Disorders Among Athletes

Some of the most frequently encountered eating disorders among athletes include Anorexia Nervosa, Bulimia Nervosa, Binge Eating Disorder, and Eating Disorder Not Otherwise Specified (EDNOS). Athletes facing these disorders often exhibit similar psychological conditions, including obsession with food and weight, body dissatisfaction, and anxiety around mealtime.

- **Anorexia Nervosa**: This disorder is characterized by severe caloric restriction, leading to unhealthy weight loss and an irrational fear of gaining weight. Athletes with anorexia may also engage in excessive exercise to control their weight, despite the negative consequences on their health and performance.
- **Bulimia Nervosa**: Bulimia involves cycles of binge eating (consuming large amounts of food in a short period) followed by compensatory behaviors to prevent weight gain, such as self-induced vomiting, laxative abuse, or excessive exercise. Athletes with bulimia typically feel a lack of control over their eating, which can be detrimental to their emotional well-being.

- **Binge Eating Disorder**: Binge Eating Disorder is characterized by recurrent episodes of binge eating without compensatory behaviors such as self-induced vomiting. Individuals with this disorder may feel intense guilt or shame after bingeing, which could adversely impact their self-esteem and athletic pursuits.
- **Eating Disorder Not Otherwise Specified (EDNOS)**: EDNOS is a term used to describe those who have some symptoms of other eating disorders but do not fully meet the criteria for a specific diagnosis. Athletes with EDNOS may still be at risk for experiencing negative consequences related to their disordered eating behaviors.

Consequences of Eating Disorders on Athletes

Eating disorders can have severe implications on an athlete's physical and mental health, leading to diminished athletic performance and possibly life-threatening consequences. Some of the most common consequences of disordered eating among athletes include:

- **Decreased muscle strength and endurance**: Inadequate caloric intake can lead to muscle wasting and a loss of strength in athletes, which translates to decreased power and endurance in their sport.
- **Reduced immune function**: Malnutrition increases the risk of illness and infection, which could result in missed training sessions, competitions, or even chronic health issues.
- **Hormonal imbalances**: Disordered eating can cause menstrual disturbances in female athletes and low testosterone levels in male athletes, both of which can negatively impact bone health and overall athletic performance.

- **Increased injury risk**: Poor nutrition and low energy availability can result in decreased bone density, making athletes more susceptible to stress fractures and other injuries.
- **Mental health challenges**: Eating disorders have been linked to increased rates of anxiety, depression, and other mental health challenges, which can significantly impact an athlete's focus, motivation, and ability to excel in their sport.

Preventing and Treating Eating Disorders in Athletes

It is crucial to address body image concerns early to prevent the development of eating disorders and promote optimal mental and physical health among athletes. Some strategies to support athletes in promoting positive body image and healthy eating habits are:

- **Education**: Ensuring that athletes, coaches, and families have access to accurate information about nutrition, body image, and the risks associated with disordered eating can be a powerful prevention tool.
- **Open communication**: Encouraging open dialogue about body image concerns and disordered eating behaviors in a supportive environment can help athletes feel more comfortable seeking help when needed.
- **Promote a positive sports culture**: Sports teams and organizations should emphasize health, wellness, and personal growth rather than just weight and appearance. Coaches and trainers can play a vital role in fostering a positive sports culture by focusing on athletes' achievements rather than emphasizing physical appearance.
- **Early intervention**: Identifying and addressing eating disorders and body image concerns as soon as

possible can prevent more severe consequences and long-term health issues. Athletes who are struggling should be encouraged to seek help from qualified professionals, such as registered dietitians, sports psychologists, or medical doctors.

In conclusion, promoting a healthy relationship with food and body image is critical to achieving optimal athletic performance and overall well-being. Understanding the nature of eating disorders, their potential impact on athletes, and strategies to prevent and treat them is essential for maintaining a healthy and thriving sports culture. By educating oneself, fostering positive communication, and promoting early intervention, we can create a sports environment conducive to the mental and physical health of all athletes.

Recognizing Eating Disorders and Promoting Positive Body Image in the Athletic Community

Eating disorders are more prevalent among athletes than in the general population, and a higher percentage of high-level athletes are affected than recreational athletes. We know now that disordered eating and poor body image can have profound consequences on an athlete's overall health and performance. In this section, we will explain the different types of eating disorders, their warning signs, and risk factors. We'll then delve into ways to promote a positive body image and create a culture of self-care and overall wellbeing within sports and athletic communities.

Types of Eating Disorders

There are several different types of eating disorders, including Anorexia Nervosa, Bulimia Nervosa, and Binge Eating Disorder. Although each disorder is distinct, they all have one thing in common: an unhealthy relationship with food and body image. Each disorder has specific signs, symptoms, and behaviors that provide clues to its presence. Knowing these signs can help identify athletes that may be in need of support and intervention.

- **Anorexia Nervosa** involves an intense fear of weight gain, distorted body image, and severe calorie restriction. People with anorexia often have a low body weight and may engage in compulsive exercise behaviors to compensate for perceived or real weight gain.
- **Bulimia Nervosa** is characterized by episodes of binge eating followed by compensatory behaviors to prevent weight gain, such as self-induced vomiting, laxative misuse, or excessive exercise. People with bulimia may maintain a normal weight or be slightly overweight, which makes this disorder challenging to recognize in athletes.
- **Binge Eating Disorder** also involves episodes of binge eating but without compensatory behaviors. Binge eating episodes are followed by feelings of guilt, shame, and self-loathing. People with binge eating disorder can be of any weight but may struggle with body dissatisfaction and a drive for thinness.

Warning Signs and Risk Factors

As you review these warning signs, bear in mind that not every athlete who exhibits these symptoms necessarily has an eating disorder. Still, it is essential to be aware of these indicators and be proactive in addressing any concerns.

- Excessive focus on body weight, shape, and size
- Frequent comments about feeling "fat" or "ugly"
- Rapid and significant weight loss (in the case of anorexia) or weight fluctuations (in bulimia and binge eating)
- Severe restriction of food intake, skipping meals, or only eating low-calorie foods
- Compulsive exercise behaviors (training beyond the requirements for their sport or continuing to exercise despite injury or illness)
- Wearing baggy clothing or layering to hide weight loss or changes in body shape
- Obsessive interest in diets, nutrition, and fad diets
- Withdrawal from or avoiding social situations involving food
- Mood swings, irritability, and depression
- Abrupt changes in athletic performance

Promoting Positive Body Image and Preventing Eating Disorders

The promotion of a healthy and positive body image is an essential component of sports culture. Here are some strategies to foster environments that promote acceptance, understanding, and self-care:

- **Emphasize the importance of function over form:** Cultivate an appreciation for what the body can do rather than what it looks like. Focus discussions on the benefits of physical activity and the importance of fueling the body for optimal performance.
- **Provide education on proper nutrition and fueling for athletes:** Ensure that your athletes are well-informed about the dietary needs specific to their sport and understand the essential role nutrition plays in performance and recovery.

- **Encourage open and honest communication:** Create an environment in which athletes feel comfortable discussing their thoughts, concerns, and anxieties related to their sport, eating habits, and body image.
- **Challenge unrealistic body ideals:** Educate athletes about the genetic factors influencing body composition and the dangers of striving for an unrealistic or unhealthy body type. Encourage athletes to appreciate the diverse range of bodies represented on their team and the unique strengths each athlete brings.
- **Monitor training and exercise loads:** Ensure that athletes are engaging in appropriate training volumes and intensity levels specific to their sport, age, and developmental level. Watch for signs of overtraining or compulsive exercise.
- **Empower athletes to set realistic goals:** Encourage goal setting that is focused on individual growth, mastery of skills, and achieving personal bests rather than interconnected with external factors such as winning or achieving a specific body weight or shape.
- **Be a role model:** Foster an environment of acceptance, understanding, and self-care. Exhibit healthy eating habits and self-esteem, and create a safe space for athletes to express their concerns and questions.

In conclusion, promoting a positive body image and understanding eating disorders in sports are essential components of an athlete's overall well-being. Making sure athletes have accurate information about nutrition, engaging in open communication, and fostering an environment that supports overall health will promote long-term success both in athletics and in life.

A. Identifying Eating Disorders and Body Image Issues in Athletes

Eating disorders and negative body image issues are relatively common among athletes and can affect individuals at any age or level of competition. However, they can be particularly prevalent in sports where body weight, physique or success is believed to be closely linked to performance. In this subsection, we will discuss the various types of eating disorders, their symptoms, potential causes, and how they can affect an athlete's mental and physical wellbeing.

1. Types of Eating Disorders

a. Anorexia Nervosa

Anorexia nervosa is characterized by self-imposed starvation, excessive weight loss, and an intense fear of gaining weight or becoming fat. Individuals with anorexia may also exhibit distorted body image, perceiving themselves as overweight even when they are underweight. Athletes with anorexia may engage in excessive exercise, restrict their caloric intake, and adopt other harmful behaviors in pursuit of an unrealistic body image or performance goal.

b. Bulimia Nervosa

Bulimia nervosa involves a cycle of binge eating and compensatory behaviors to prevent weight gain, such as self-induced vomiting, misuse of laxatives or diuretics, fasting, or excessive exercise. This cycle is typically driven by feelings of guilt or shame about binge eating, and the desire to regain control over one's body and weight. Athletes with bulimia may experience fluctuations in weight, and struggle with body image dissatisfaction and low self-esteem.

c. Binge-Eating Disorder

Binge-eating disorder is characterized by recurrent episodes of eating unusually large amounts of food in a short period of time, often accompanied by feelings of loss of control, guilt, and embarrassment. Unlike bulimia, binge-eating disorder does not involve regular compensatory behaviors to prevent weight gain. As a result, individuals with this disorder may be of normal weight, overweight, or obese. Athletes with binge-eating disorder may struggle with their relationship with food and body image and may be more vulnerable to weight-related health issues or injury.

d. Other Specified Feeding or Eating Disorder (OSFED)

OSFED is a category of eating disorders that do not meet the full criteria for anorexia nervosa, bulimia nervosa, or binge-eating disorder, but still cause significant emotional and physical distress. OSFED can manifest in diverse ways, such as purging disorder, night eating syndrome, or atypical anorexia nervosa. Athletes with OSFED may experience a range of symptoms and challenges depending on their unique presentation of the disorder, and it can still interfere significantly with their performance and overall wellbeing.

2. Symptoms, Warning Signs, and Consequences

Recognizing the symptoms and warning signs of an eating disorder is essential for early intervention and treatment, which can prevent lasting physical and emotional harm. Some common signs of an eating disorder in athletes include:

- Rapid, unexplained weight loss or weight gain
- Obsession with food, diet, and body weight or shape
- Avoidance of social situations or events involving food
- Using the bathroom immediately after eating or during meals
- Signs of self-induced vomiting, such as swollen cheeks, abrasions on the knuckles, or dental issues
- Exercising excessively, even when injured or exhausted
- Emotional withdrawal, irritability, or depression
- Fatigue or difficulty concentrating

It's important to note that an athlete may not exhibit all of these signs, and the presence of these signs does not automatically indicate an eating disorder. However, understanding these warning signs can help identify possible concerns that should be carefully evaluated by a professional.

The consequences of eating disorders for athletes can be severe, including impaired athletic performance, increased risk for injury, nutritional deficiencies, electrolyte imbalances, hormonal disturbances, weakened immune function, and mental health challenges.

3. Causes and Risk Factors

Eating disorders are complex and often arise from a combination of genetic, psychological, social, and cultural factors. In athletes, specific factors that may increase their vulnerability to developing an eating disorder or negative body image include:

- Pressure to maintain a specific body weight, size, or shape for their sport

- Coaching or team culture that emphasizes weight or appearance as essential for success
- Chronic dieting or restrictive eating patterns
- History of weight cycling, yo-yo dieting, or disordered eating
- Sports that emphasize aesthetics or require form-fitting uniforms
- Perfectionism or highly competitive nature
- Low self-esteem or poor body image
- A history of trauma, abuse, or mental health issues

In the next subsection, we will explore proactive strategies and interventions that can be implemented by athletes, coaches, and support teams to promote healthy relationships with food, body image, and sport. This will involve creating an inclusive and supportive environment, addressing risk factors, and ensuring early intervention and treatment for those who may be struggling with eating disorders or body image concerns.

Copyrights and Content Disclaimer:

AI-Assisted Content Disclaimer:
The content of this book has been generated with the assistance of artificial intelligence (AI) language models like CHatGPT and Llama. While efforts have been made to ensure the accuracy and relevance of the information provided, the author and publisher make no warranties or guarantees regarding the completeness, reliability, or suitability of the content for any specific purpose. The AI-generated content may contain errors, inaccuracies, or outdated information, and readers should exercise caution and independently verify any information before relying on it. The author and publisher shall not be held responsible for any consequences arising from the use of or reliance on the AI-generated content in this book.

General Disclaimer:
We use content-generating tools for creating this book and source a large amount of the material from text-generation tools. We make financial material and data available through our Services. In order to do so we rely on a variety of sources to gather this information. We believe these to be reliable, credible, and accurate sources. However, there may be times when the information is incorrect.
WE MAKE NO CLAIMS OR REPRESENTATIONS AS TO THE ACCURACY, COMPLETENESS, OR TRUTH OF ANY MATERIAL CONTAINED ON OUR book. NOR WILL WE BE LIABLE FOR ANY ERRORS INACCURACIES OR OMISSIONS, AND SPECIFICALLY DISCLAIMS ANY IMPLIED WARRANTIES OR MERCHANTABILITY OR FITNESS FOR ANY PARTICULAR PURPOSE AND SHALL IN NO EVENT BE LIABLE FOR ANY LOSS OF PROFIT OR ANY OTHER COMMERCIAL OR PROPERTY DAMAGE, INCLUDING BUT NOT LIMITED TO SPECIAL, INCIDENTAL, CONSEQUENTIAL, OR OTHER DAMAGES; OR FOR

DELAYS IN THE CONTENT OR TRANSMISSION OF THE DATA
ON OUR book, OR THAT THE BOOK WILL ALWAYS BE
AVAILABLE.

In addition to the above, it is important to note that language
models like ChatGPT are based on deep learning techniques
and have been trained on vast amounts of text data to generate
human-like text. This text data includes a variety of sources
such as books, articles, websites, and much more. This training
process allows the model to learn patterns and relationships
within the text and generate outputs that are coherent and
contextually appropriate.

Language models like ChatGPT can be used in a variety of
applications, including but not limited to, customer service,
content creation, and language translation. In customer
service, for example, language models can be used to answer
customer inquiries quickly and accurately, freeing up human
agents to handle more complex tasks. In content creation,
language models can be used to generate articles, summaries,
and captions, saving time and effort for content creators. In
language translation, language models can assist in translating
text from one language to another with high accuracy, helping
to break down language barriers.

It's important to keep in mind, however, that while language
models have made great strides in generating human-like text,
they are not perfect. There are still limitations to the model's
understanding of the context and meaning of the text, and it
may generate outputs that are incorrect or offensive. As such,
it's important to use language models with caution and always
verify the accuracy of the outputs generated by the model.

Financial Disclaimer

This book is dedicated to helping you understand the world of
online investing, removing any fears you may have about

getting started and helping you choose good investments. Our goal is to help you take control of your financial well-being by delivering a solid financial education and responsible investing strategies. However, the information contained on this book and in our services is for general information and educational purposes only. It is not intended as a substitute for legal, commercial and/or financial advice from a licensed professional. The business of online investing is a complicated matter that requires serious financial due diligence for each investment in order to be successful. You are strongly advised to seek the services of qualified, competent professionals prior to engaging in any investment that may impact you finances. This information is provided by this book, including how it was made, collectively referred to as the "Services."

Be Careful With Your Money. Only use strategies that you both understand the potential risks of and are comfortable taking. It is your responsibility to invest wisely and to safeguard your personal and financial information.

We believe we have a great community of investors looking to achieve and help each other achieve financial success through investing. Accordingly we encourage people to comment on our blog and possibly in the future our forum. Many people will contribute in this matter, however, there will be times when people provide misleading, deceptive or incorrect information, unintentionally or otherwise.

You should NEVER rely upon any information or opinions you read on this book, or any book that we may link to. The information you read here and in our services should be used as a launching point for your OWN RESEARCH into various companies and investing strategies so that you can make an informed decision about where and how to invest your money.

WE DO NOT GUARANTEE THE VERACITY, RELIABILITY OR COMPLETENESS OF ANY INFORMATION PROVIDED IN THE COMMENTS, FORUM OR OTHER PUBLIC AREAS OF THE book OR IN ANY HYPERLINK APPEARING ON OUR book.

Our Services are provided to help you to understand how to make good investment and personal financial decisions for yourself. You are solely responsible for the investment decisions you make. We will not be responsible for any errors or omissions on the book including in articles or postings, for hyperlinks embedded in messages, or for any results obtained from the use of such information. Nor, will we be liable for any loss or damage, including consequential damages, if any, caused by a reader's reliance on any information obtained through the use of our Services. Please do not use our book If you do not accept self-responsibility for your actions.

The U.S. Securities and Exchange Commission, (SEC), has published additional information on Cyberfraud to help you recognize and combat it effectively. You can also get additional help about online investment schemes and how to avoid them at the following books:http://www.sec.gov and http://www.finra.org, and http://www.nasaa.org these are each organizations set-up to help protect online investors.

If you choose ignore our advice and do not do independent research of the various industries, companies, and stocks, you intend to invest in and rely solely on information, "tips," or opinions found on our book – you agree that you have made a conscious, personal decision of your own free will and will not try to hold us responsible for the results thereof under any circumstance. The Services offered herein is not for the purpose of acting as your personal investment advisor. We do not know all the relevant facts about you and/or your individual needs, and we do not represent or claim that any of our Services are suitable for your needs. You should seek a registered investment advisor if you are looking for personalized advice.

Links to Other Sites. You will also be able to link to other books from time to time, through our Site. We do not have any control over the content or actions of the books we link to and will not be liable for anything that occurs in connection with the use of such books. The inclusion of any links, unless otherwise expressly stated, should not be seen as an endorsement or recommendation of that book or the views expressed therein. You, and only you, are responsible for doing your own due diligence on any book prior to doing any business with them.

Liability Disclaimers and Limitations: Under no circumstances, including but not limited to negligence, will we, nor our partners if any, or any of our affiliates, be held responsible or liable, directly or indirectly, for any loss or damage, whatsoever arising out of, or in connection with, the use of our Services, including without limitation, direct, indirect, consequential, unexpected, special, exemplary or other damages that may result, including but not limited to economic loss, injury, illness or death or any other type of loss or damage, or unexpected or adverse reactions to suggestions contained herein or otherwise caused or alleged to have been caused to you in connection with your use of any advice, goods or services you receive on the Site, regardless of the source, or any other book that you may have visited via links from our book, even if advised of the possibility of such damages.

Applicable law may not allow the limitation or exclusion of liability or incidental or consequential damages (including but not limited to lost data), so the above limitation or exclusion may not apply to you. However, in no event shall the total liability to you by us for all damages, losses, and causes of action (whether in contract, tort, or otherwise) exceed the amount paid by you to us, if any, for the use of our Services, if any. And by using our Site you expressly agree not to try to hold us liable for any consequences that result based on your use of our Services or the information provided therein, at any time, or for any reason, regardless of the circumstances.

Specific Results Disclaimer. We are dedicated to helping you take control of your financial well-being through education and investment. We provide strategies, opinions, resources and other Services that are specifically designed to cut through the noise and hype to help you make better personal finance and investment decisions. However, there is no way to guarantee any strategy or technique to be 100% effective, as results will vary by individual, and the effort and commitment they make toward achieving their goal. And, unfortunately we don't know you. Therefore, in using and/or purchasing our services you expressly agree that the results you receive from the use of those Services are solely up to you. In addition, you also expressly agree that all risks of use and any consequences of such use shall be borne exclusively by you. And that you will not to try to hold us liable at any time, or for any reason, regardless of the circumstances.

As stipulated by law, we can not and do not make any guarantees about your ability to achieve any particular results by using any Service purchased through our book. Nothing on this page, our book, or any of our services is a promise or guarantee of results, including that you will make any particular amount of money or, any money at all, you also understand, that all investments come with some risk and you may actually lose money while investing. Accordingly, any results stated on our book, in the form of testimonials, case studies or otherwise are illustrative of concepts only and should not be considered average results, or promises for actual or future performance.

tolerance, and the ability to consistently apply the strategies and techniques discussed.

Copyright Notice: All rights reserved. No part of this publication may be reproduced, distributed, or transmitted in any form or by any means, including photocopying, recording, or other electronic or mechanical methods, without the prior written permission of the publisher, except in the case of brief quotations embodied in critical reviews and certain other noncommercial uses permitted by copyright law.

Trademarks: All product names, logos, and brands mentioned in this book are property of their respective owners. Use of these names, logos, and brands does not imply endorsement by or affiliation with their respective owners.